NATIONAL ACADEMIES
Sciences
Engineering
Medicine

NATIONAL ACADEMIES PRESS
Washington, DC

Living with ALS

Alan I. Leshner, Rebecca A. English, and Joe Alper, *Editors*

Committee on Amyotrophic Lateral Sclerosis:
Accelerating Treatments and Improving Quality of Life

Board on Health Care Services

Board on Health Sciences Policy

Health and Medicine Division

Consensus Study Report

NATIONAL ACADEMIES PRESS 500 Fifth Street, NW Washington, DC 20001

This activity was supported by a contract between the National Academy of Sciences and the National Institute of Neurological Disorders and Stroke, National Institutes of Health (contract number HHSN263201800029I, task order 75N98022F00011). Any opinions, findings, conclusions, or recommendations expressed in this publication do not necessarily reflect the views of any organization or agency that provided support for the project.

International Standard Book Number-13: 978-0-309-71801-1
International Standard Book Number-10: 0-309-71801-5
Digital Object Identifier: https://doi.org/10.17226/27739

This publication is available from the National Academies Press, 500 Fifth Street, NW, Keck 360, Washington, DC 20001; (800) 624-6242 or (202) 334-3313; http://www.nap.edu.

Suggested citation: National Academies of Sciences, Engineering, and Medicine. 2024. *Living with ALS*. Washington, DC: The National Academies Press. https://doi.org/10.17226/27739.

The **National Academy of Sciences** was established in 1863 by an Act of Congress, signed by President Lincoln, as a private, nongovernmental institution to advise the nation on issues related to science and technology. Members are elected by their peers for outstanding contributions to research. Dr. Marcia McNutt is president.

The **National Academy of Engineering** was established in 1964 under the charter of the National Academy of Sciences to bring the practices of engineering to advising the nation. Members are elected by their peers for extraordinary contributions to engineering. Dr. John L. Anderson is president.

The **National Academy of Medicine** (formerly the Institute of Medicine) was established in 1970 under the charter of the National Academy of Sciences to advise the nation on medical and health issues. Members are elected by their peers for distinguished contributions to medicine and health. Dr. Victor J. Dzau is president.

The three Academies work together as the **National Academies of Sciences, Engineering, and Medicine** to provide independent, objective analysis and advice to the nation and conduct other activities to solve complex problems and inform public policy decisions. The National Academies also encourage education and research, recognize outstanding contributions to knowledge, and increase public understanding in matters of science, engineering, and medicine.

Learn more about the National Academies of Sciences, Engineering, and Medicine at **www.nationalacademies.org**.

ANANTHA SHEKHAR, Senior Vice Chancellor for the Health Sciences, John and Gertrude Petersen Dean, School of Medicine, University of Pittsburgh

MINDY UHRLAUB, Author and familial ALS activist; member, Peer Mentor Team and Familial ALS Team at I AM ALS; founding member, Genetic ALS & FTD: End the Legacy

Study Staff

REBECCA A. ENGLISH, Study Director
ASHLEY BOLOGNA, Senior Program Assistant
LYLE CARRERA, Research Associate
SHARYL NASS, Senior Director, Board on Health Care Services
CLARE STROUD, Senior Director, Board on Health Sciences Policy

Consultants

JOE ALPER, Science writer
SARAH LUNSFORD, Public engagement consultant

Reviewers

This Consensus Study Report was reviewed in draft form by individuals chosen for their diverse perspectives and technical expertise. The purpose of this independent review is to provide candid and critical comments that will assist the National Academies of Sciences, Engineering, and Medicine in making each published report as sound as possible and to ensure that it meets the institutional standards for quality, objectivity, evidence, and responsiveness to the study charge. The review comments and draft manuscript remain confidential to protect the integrity of the deliberative process.

We thank the following individuals for their review of this report:

JINSY ANDREWS, Columbia University
LORA CLAWSON, Johns Hopkins University School of Medicine
MARY CATHERINE COLLET, Independent ALS advocate
KULDIP DAVE, ALS Association
GREGG GONSALVES, Yale University
JOHN HANSEN-FLASCHEN, University of Pennsylvania
KATHLEEN U. HOLT, Center for Medicare Advocacy
COLLIN HOVINGA, Critical Path Institute
STORY LANDIS, National Institute of Neurological Disorders and
    Stroke (retired)
NANCY LEAMOND, AARP
JEAN SWIDLER, Genetic ALS & FTD: End the Legacy
NETA ZACH, Takeda
BERNIE ZIPPRICH, Healthcare innovation expert and person living
    with ALS

Although the reviewers listed above provided many constructive comments and suggestions, they were not asked to endorse the conclusions or recommendations of this report nor did they see the final draft before its release. The review of this report was overseen by **JONATHAN M. SAMET,** Colorado School of Public Health, and **DAN G. BLAZER II,** Duke University School of Medicine. They were responsible for making certain that an independent examination of this report was carried out in accordance with the standards of the National Academies and that all review comments were carefully considered. Responsibility for the final content rests entirely with the authoring committee and the National Academies.

Acknowledgments

The committee and project staff extend their gratitude to the many people and organizations who were critical in supporting and informing the committee's work. This study was sponsored by the National Institutes of Health (NIH) and, in particular, was supported by the National Institute of Neurological Diseases and Stroke (NINDS). The committee thanks NIH and NINDS for their support, and the committee thanks Congress for initiating this important study.

People with amyotrophic lateral sclerosis (ALS), their caregivers and family members, representatives of ALS nonprofit organizations, researchers, and clinicians graciously offered their expertise and perspectives throughout the study process. This information was not only useful but also courageous, heartfelt, and inspiring. The committee heard from many people in different ways throughout the study and would like to extend its appreciation to each.

Over the course of its meetings, the committee heard from many people who shared their stories about ALS. This allowed the committee to center their work in the real-world lived experiences of those living with and affected by this disease, as well as to gain valuable insight as to the challenges and opportunities faced by those who fight against ALS in their daily lives, at labs or clinics, and alongside countless community organizations. The committee thanks the many participants in its public sessions: Lori Banker-Horner, James Berry, Sunny Brous, Katrina Byrd, Nora Capocci, Blair Casey, Jim Clingman, Sylvia Clingman, Cathy Collet, Norah Crossnohere, Penny Dacks, Dan Doctoroff, Sonya Elling, Ron Faretra, Albert Faro, Sarah Fontaine, Renee Golden, John

Hansen-Flaschen, Bob Hebron, Terry Heiman-Patterson, Colleen Hoarty, Collin Hovinga, Justin Ichida, Vanessa Jackson, Asia Jami, Desiree Galvez Kessler, Lisa Latts, Ashley Lee, Melanie Lendnal, Joanne Lynn, Paul Mehta, Paul Melmeyer, Indu Navar, Siobhan Pandya, Juliet Pierce, Terri Postma, Kristin Rankin, Julian Rodriguez, Bruce Rosenblum, Paul Seifert, Jean Swidler, Neil Thakur, Fernando Vieira, and William Woods.

The committee also benefited from the perspectives of six individuals appointed as lived experience consultants (volunteers). The lived experience consultants provided reflections on some excerpts of draft report text between January and March 2024. The committee expresses its gratitude to Michael Cosgray, Desiree Galvez Kessler, Bernadine A. Okeke, Ann Oliff, Kristin Rankin, and Julian (Jules) Rodriguez for their participation in the study process as lived experience consultants.

The committee also thanks Sarah Lunsford, who served as a consultant to organize many of these public engagement opportunities.

The staff of the National Academies of Sciences, Engineering, and Medicine contributed in many ways throughout the study process. The committee extends its sincerest gratitude to the study team for their hard work and dedication throughout this project: Rebecca A. English, Lyle Carrera, and Ashley Bologna. The committee is grateful for the many staff within the Health and Medicine Division who provided support for the project. Special thanks are extended to Christie Bell, senior financial business partner; Lori Brenig, editorial projects coordinator; and Mark Goodin for his editorial assistance in preparing the report.

Contents

Boxes, Figures, and Tables

TABLES

Acronyms and Abbreviations

ACT for ALS	Accelerating Access to Critical Therapies for ALS Act
AHRQ	Agency for Healthcare Research and Quality
ALL ALS	Access for ALL in ALS Clinical Research Consortium
ALS	amyotrophic lateral sclerosis
ALSA	ALS Association
ALSFRS-R	Revised Amyotrophic Lateral Sclerosis Functional Rating Scale
AMP ALS	Accelerating Medicines Partnership for ALS
BCI	brain–computer interface
CDC	Centers for Disease Control and Prevention
CFF	Cystic Fibrosis Foundation
CFFPR	Cystic Fibrosis Foundation Patient Registry
CMS	Centers for Medicare & Medicaid Services
CP-RND	Critical Path for Rare Neurodegenerative Diseases
DME	durable medical equipment
DVT	deep venous thrombosis
FDA	U.S. Food and Drug Administration
FNIH	Foundation for the National Institutes of Health
FQHC	Federally Qualified Health Center
FTD	frontotemporal dementia

GDNF	glial cell line-derived neurotrophic factor
GINA	Genetic Information Nondiscrimination Act
GUIDE	Guiding an Improved Dementia Experience
HHS	U.S. Department of Health and Human Services
HMV	home mechanical ventilation
MDA	Muscular Dystrophy Association
MGH	Massachusetts General Hospital
MND	motor neuron disease
NCI	National Cancer Institute
NCRI	Neurological Clinical Research Institute
NEALS	Northeast ALS Consortium
NeuroNEXT	Network for Excellence in Neuroscience Clinical Trials
NfL	neurofilament light chain
NIH	National Institutes of Health
NINDS	National Institute of Neurological Disorders and Stroke
NIV	noninvasive ventilation
PFT	pulmonary function test
Pre-fALS	Pre-symptomatic Familial ALS Study
PRO-ACT	Pooled Resource Open-Access ALS Clinical Trials Database
SSDI	Social Security Disability Insurance
VA	U.S. Department of Veterans Affairs

Preface

Amyotrophic lateral sclerosis (ALS) is a terrible, inevitably fatal disease. Receiving a diagnosis of ALS is devastating for people living with ALS, their families, and their caregivers. Dealing with this illness requires a complex array of medical and support service interventions, and the intensity of care required increases exponentially over time. This report lays out an agenda that, if implemented, would provide greater and more equitable access to state-of-the-art multidisciplinary care, accelerate the development of more effective treatments, improve the quality of life and health of those individuals suffering from the illness both now and in the future, and provide better support for their families and caregivers. Implementing this agenda would go far toward the goal set in the committee's charge of making ALS a livable disease within a decade.

This consensus report is the product of a committee of scientific and clinical experts from a variety of fields, as well as individuals living with the disease and people at clear risk for developing it. In addition, the committee met with a variety of other people living with the illness and asked them to reflect on the relevance of the committee's thinking and its potential recommendations. Including these individuals in our work helped greatly to ground the committee's work in real-life experiences and, I believe, significantly improved both the quality of this report and the appropriateness of its recommendations.

As discussed in the report, the committee was aware that at the same time it was working on this project, many other, often parallel projects with similar goals were ongoing. We tried to remain cognizant of those efforts in framing our report and recommendations so as to avoid inadvertent conflicts or excessive duplication in strategies for accomplishing our shared goals.

Achieving the vision underlying this report will require commitment and leadership from many different stakeholders. Some of the report's recommendations require substantial resources, but their impacts will be great for the more than 30,000 individuals living with ALS and the thousands more who are at clear risk of developing the disease. The steps recommended here include developing a comprehensive multidisciplinary care and research network that would do much to ensure substantially more equitable access to state-of-the-art care for all individuals with ALS, reduce unacceptably long delays in receiving an accurate diagnosis, significantly expand the research infrastructure needed to develop new and improved treatments and support services, and explore new ways to help finance appropriate care and supports. As with all endeavors with grand goals, achieving the agenda laid out here will not only require substantial resources and leadership from a variety of stakeholders, but these diverse groups will have to come together with a common focus and consistent messages about what is needed to make real progress against this dreaded disease.

I am extremely grateful to my colleagues on the National Academies of Sciences, Engineering, and Medicine committee that authored this report. It was both an honor and a pleasure to work with them all. I also want to express, on behalf of the whole committee, our gratitude to the exceptionally competent and dedicated staff of the National Academies, led by the study director, Rebecca English, and the many others cited in the acknowledgments.

Alan I. Leshner, *Chair*
Committee on Amyotrophic Lateral Sclerosis: Accelerating
Treatments and Improving Quality of Life

Summary

Amyotrophic lateral sclerosis (ALS) is a rapidly progressive, fatal neurological disease for which there are no treatments that stop or reverse disease progression. At least 30,000 individuals in the United States have ALS at any given time. The pathological hallmark of ALS is progressive degeneration of motor neurons that causes a gradual loss of motor functions, but no two people with ALS will experience the disease in the same way or have their disease progress at the same rate.

Approximately two-thirds of individuals with ALS initially experience effects in the muscles of the hands, forearms, calves, and feet. This form of ALS is called limb-onset ALS. The other one-third of patients first experience weakness in the muscles around the mouth and throat and develop what is called bulbar-onset ALS. Over time, these symptoms progress toward other areas of the body until all muscle groups are paralyzed. People with ALS often find motor tasks such as walking, eating, and interacting with objects increasingly difficult as their disease progresses, and many then require assistance with day-to-day activities. Death usually results from respiratory failure when the muscles responsible for breathing become paralyzed. People living with ALS typically experience respiratory failure within 2 to 5 years of when symptoms first appear. Approximately 10 to 20 percent of ALS patients survive longer than 10 years and this is typically seen in people with younger-onset ALS. ALS subtype affects survival, as do genetics and cognitive involvement.

ALS is a multisystem disease with a high prevalence of secondary symptoms, including fatigue, pain, insomnia, anxiety, depression, and shortness of breath. The effect of secondary symptoms affecting quality of life is not as well recognized.

Sporadic ALS occurs randomly in individuals without a family history of ALS and accounts for approximately 90 percent of all cases. Familial ALS refers to individuals with ALS who have a known family history of the disease. Seventy percent of individuals with familial ALS are carriers of known ALS-associated gene mutations. Research has identified close to 50 genes associated with ALS when mutated, with additional gene variants considered to be risk factors of ALS disease manifestation.

Research has linked contributions from a variety of environmental exposures to the development of sporadic ALS. These include exposure to pesticides and air pollution, being a veteran or working in occupations such as agriculture and painting, and exposure to repeat physical trauma.

NATIONAL ACADEMIES STUDY PROCESS

In response to the devastating nature of ALS for individuals and their families, Congress, in the Consolidated Appropriations Act of 2022, directed the National Institutes of Health (NIH) to commission a study by the National Academies of Sciences, Engineering, and Medicine (the National Academies) to identify and recommend actions for the public, private, and nonprofit sectors to undertake that would make ALS a livable disease within a decade. The National Institute of Neurological Disorders and Stroke (NINDS) contracted with the National Academies to address the statement of task (see Box 1-1 in Chapter 1).

The National Academies established a committee of 18 volunteer experts with the experience and skills to accomplish the statement of task.[1] The committee included individuals with expertise in neurology, rehabilitation, pulmonary, and primary care; translational ALS and frontotemporal dementia (FTD) research; health law and policy; ethics; public health; health care financing; nursing and long-term care; and therapeutic development and regulatory pathways, as well individuals with ALS lived experience. The committee considered the scientific literature on ALS and listened to and carefully considered the perspectives of people affected by ALS. This included perspectives of people living with ALS, caregivers, family members, and people with a genetic risk of developing ALS.

---

[1] See https://www.nationalacademies.org/about for a detailed overview of the National Academies and see https://www.nationalacademies.org/about/our-study-process for an overview of the National Academies' study process (accessed June 10, 2024).

LIVING WITH ALS TODAY

In the committee's own discussions, and in discussions with people living with ALS, the committee realized that making the disease "livable" has two important, primary dimensions: (1) increasing the effectiveness of treatment, with the goal of managing symptoms, increasing longevity and ultimately finding a cure; and (2) increasing the quality of life, as measured by the level of satisfaction and enjoyment experienced by people with ALS. This means that ALS is livable when an individual diagnosed with ALS or at genetic risk of developing ALS can survive, thrive, and live a long, meaningful life while meeting the medical, psychosocial, and economic challenges of the disease. Guaranteeing equitable access to high-quality multidisciplinary care for all individuals, regardless of socioeconomic status or geographical location, is of paramount importance. This would include providing affordable and equitable access to physical, occupational, speech, respiratory, and behavioral therapies; nutritional support; durable medical equipment (DME), such as electric wheelchairs and home ventilators; and palliative care, all without having to prove present or future necessity, given the diagnosis of ALS. Eliminating the substantial delay many people with ALS experience in getting a clear diagnosis is also critically important, both to start multidisciplinary care as soon as possible and to alleviate the substantial emotional burden that comes with waiting and uncertainty while circling around a diagnosis. Reducing diagnostic delay will require, in part, better educating primary care physicians and general neurologists about ALS and its many presentations.

Other issues that make life harder for individuals affected by ALS include:

- *Insurance barriers*: People with ALS can face challenges in acquiring medically indicated equipment, technology, and therapeutics and dealing with an often-convoluted system for obtaining prior authorizations.
- *Inadequate home services*: There is a serious challenge in accessing high-quality, affordable home health services for the complex and evolving needs of people with ALS.
- *Inadequate access to respiratory care*: Despite strong evidence that proactive respiratory management prolongs survival and improves quality of life, barriers remain to delivering optimal clinical respiratory care for people living with ALS.
- *High out-of-pocket costs*: The out-of-pocket costs for individuals with ALS and their families vary greatly—individuals with ALS who receive care through the Department of Veterans Affairs are spared financial devastation whereas many individuals with ALS

who have private insurance need to seek other financial support for home modifications or services and devices they need to make the disease more livable. ALS was the most common neurological condition that users created campaigns for on GoFundMe, a crowd-sourced fundraising platform.

- *Caregivers*: The physical, emotional, and financial demands of caring for someone with ALS are substantial and can lead to depression, anxiety, burnout, and other impairments.

Providing Multidisciplinary Care Is Key

The committee believes that every individual living with ALS deserves early and continuous access to multidisciplinary,[2] state-of-the-art care to help them lead longer lives, remain functionally independent, and optimize overall quality of life. Multidisciplinary clinics provide coordinated, team-based management across multiple medical and allied health specialties and serve as a one-stop shop for complex multisystem diseases, such as ALS. However, there is no definitive count of the number of people living with ALS today who receive evidence-based standard of care at a multidisciplinary clinic but one estimate from the ALS Association suggests that it is at best about half of the population.[3] A multidisciplinary care clinic serves as a single site for many services for people living with ALS, confirming diagnosis, initiating and monitoring therapies, providing medications and assistive technology devices, and managing multisystem symptoms. A multidisciplinary care clinic also directly provides or provides connections to specialized health and supportive services to track disease progression, improve quality of life, and prolong functional independence. A multidisciplinary care clinic may also provide palliative care services for individualized advanced care planning based on ALS disease progression.

---

[2] As stated in Chapter 2, the committee notes that *interdisciplinary*, rather than *multidisciplinary*, is the more accurate term because interdisciplinary denotes that the various disciplines are coordinated toward a common and coherent approach, while multidisciplinary refers to the addition of the competencies of multiple professionals who stay within the boundaries of their fields. The Veterans Health Administration refers to the ALS interdisciplinary team in its directive on providing ALS care to veterans. The committee has chosen to use *multidisciplinary* in the report because it is the more widely used term.

[3] In an October 18, 2023, letter to the committee from the ALS Association, it is stated: "Although multidisciplinary ALS care can add nine months of life, it is woefully underfunded and often difficult to deliver. Only about half the people served at ALS Certified Treatment Centers of Excellence receive this well-established, evidence-based standard of care."

In this report the committee offers recommendations in the following four domains that, if implemented, would make ALS a more livable disease within a decade.

1. Short-term actions to remove barriers for people with ALS to receive care and services that improve quality of life (Recommendations 3-1 to 3-5).
2. Longer-term actions to build a sustainable, integrated, and coordinated system of ALS care and research (Recommendations 4-1 to 4-4).
3. Actions to improve epidemiological data, accelerate research and therapeutic development, and advance understanding of what works best in ALS care (Recommendations 5-1 to 5-4).
4. Actions to advance ALS prevention research and ultimately stop the disease from developing in at-risk populations (Recommendations 6-1 and 6-2).

Actions That Are Feasible Immediately and Would Have an Important Effect on Livability

The following short-term actions are recommended by the committee to make ALS a livable disease (Recommendations 3-1 to 3-5):

Recommendation 3-1: Facilitate expedited access to and coverage of essential ALS medical and support services.

The Centers for Medicare & Medicaid Services (CMS) and private insurers should act quickly to enable expedited access to the following essential ALS medical and support services:

a. Provide coverage for home-based and outpatient physical and other support services for persons with ALS as necessary, of the type and duration needed by persons with ALS, even if services are occurring concomitantly. Congress should grant CMS the authority to provide concomitant services at home and as an outpatient for progressive, neurodegenerative diseases such as ALS.

b. Commit to expedited (within 72 hours) responses to prior authorization requests for all therapies, durable medical equipment, assistive technologies, and services for persons with ALS.

c. Do not deny services for persons with ALS based on failure to show functional improvement, given the progressive nature of the illness.

d. Establish a call center for persons living with ALS, and possibly other rare diseases, and their caregivers to report challenges in receiving care and services.

   e. Work with ALS organizations and persons living with ALS and
       their families to develop a "Know Your Rights" document that
       describes Medicare, Medicaid, and private insurance require-
       ments and empowers individuals living with ALS to combat
       misinformation and improper denial of services.

Recommendation 3-2: Enable all persons with ALS to access and make full use of ALS care.

Congress should act quickly to enable all persons with ALS to access timely, specialty ALS care by doing the following:

   a. Expand the status of ALS as a qualifying condition for
       Medicare coverage, such that persons with ALS are eligible
       for Medicare coverage regardless of age, employment his-
       tory, or other criteria influencing Medicare or Social Security
       Disability Insurance eligibility.
   b. Require reimbursement of multidisciplinary ALS care under
       a bundled payment method commensurate with the services
       provided.

Recommendation 3-3: Provide centralized resources for people with ALS to receive support for needs not otherwise accessible or covered by insurance. ALS nonprofit organizations and patient-serving associations should collaborate to create and maintain centralized resources to guide people with ALS and their caregivers to organizations and funding mechanisms that can provide financial support for needs not otherwise accessible to them or covered by Medicare, Medicaid, and private insurance. These might include such things as mental health services, modifications to home environments, securing equipment and assistive technologies, and transportation.

Recommendation 3-4: Address the needs of unpaid caregivers.

Congress, the Centers for Medicare & Medicaid Services (CMS), private insurers, and ALS organizations should address the needs of unpaid caregivers, including respite care, reimbursement for care-giving, and mental and other health support services, including the following:

   a. National and local ALS nonprofits should collaborate to
       develop a priority list of caregiver needs to inform collec-
       tive advocacy efforts of national ALS nonprofits. This could
       be accompanied by a guide for ALS caregivers on what to
       expect through the course of disease and identify resources,

which would be used by all national nonprofits and updated collaboratively.

b. Congress should provide financial support for caregivers by amending the tax code to provide a tax credit that could be used by caregivers for individuals living with ALS, as well as all progressive neurodegenerative diseases to alleviate the financial burden of providing unpaid care. Congress should also provide other types of financial relief for caregivers, including allowing them to apply health savings account or flexible saving account funds to caring for a parent or parent-in-law.

c. CMS should ensure legally covered services for home health aides are accessible.

d. CMS should expand tests of payment and service delivery models, such as the Guiding an Improved Dementia Experience model for people with dementia and their caregivers, to include ALS, or create new programs specifically designed to support persons with ALS and their unpaid caregivers. These tests should include:

  • Stipends paid directly to caregivers on an at least a monthly basis,
  • Reimbursing persons with ALS and their caregivers for accessing mental health counseling and psychotherapy via video telehealth (across state lines), and
  • Access to high-quality respite care services.

Recommendation 3-5: Enable access to respiratory devices and services for people with ALS.

The Centers for Medicare & Medicaid Services (CMS) and private insurers should immediately align coverage of respiratory devices and services for persons with ALS with the current standard of care. CMS and private insurers should also develop reimbursement models that allow respiratory professionals to provide high-quality, longitudinal respiratory care in the home of a person with ALS.

BUILDING THE IDEAL ALS CARE DELIVERY SYSTEM

Today, there is notable variation across clinics in the quality and consistency of care individuals with ALS receive, including prescribing of standard-of-care therapeutics, use of noninvasive ventilation, use of off-label supplements and medications, clinical trial participation, and access to investigational therapies via expanded access protocols. Making ALS a livable disease requires diagnosing individuals earlier and initiating evidence-based multidisciplinary care by ALS specialists immediately and continuously. At the same time, because of the progressive nature of the disease that makes travel difficult, individuals living with ALS need access to multidisciplinary care at a geographically accessible location in their communities or via telehealth to ensure continuous access to care services throughout the illness. Simply proliferating the number of stand-alone ALS clinics will not solve the issue of earlier referral because the current clinic system is not integrated or coordinated. What is feasible is to build a reimagined, inclusive, and integrated care and research system for people living with ALS, building on what already exists, that comprises three care settings: (1) Community-Based ALS Centers, (2) Regional ALS Centers, and (3) Comprehensive ALS Care and Research Centers. This new system, modeled after "hub-and-spoke" systems of care and research for cancer and stroke, is designed to fill gaps in access to ALS care and research across the United States. Each care setting in the network would provide defined clinical care services and research capabilities and be accountable for achieving quality metrics.

Every person with ALS and their family will be able to use all three care settings to meet their needs for specialized care and research services at a geographically convenient location. The reimagined ALS care system will build on and strengthen the preexisting ALS Association– and Muscular Dystrophy Association–certified multidisciplinary clinic systems, centralizing oversight to ensure care quality, provide additional infrastructures to collect population health data, and coordinate care across settings. This system will encourage innovative approaches to bringing care to people with ALS such as expanded telehealth services, house call visits, and satellite clinics.

The resulting highly integrated system of care should more easily reach underrepresented and underserved people living with ALS and those living in remote areas of the United States and all U.S. territories. Today, there are many non-ALS-trained neurologists providing care to people living with ALS in general neurology or general neuromuscular clinics who could be integrated into the new ALS care system under the guidance of Comprehensive ALS Care and Research Centers. This would expand the number of general neurology and neuromuscular clinics within the ALS care and research system, enhancing access to care and reducing the time to diagnosis.

The committee notes that the U.S. Department of Veterans Affairs (VA) has demonstrated an exemplary system of ALS care that is interdisciplinary, proactive, and patient-centric. One unique and important feature of the VA model is that veterans with ALS are largely spared the substantial financial burdens related to ongoing care and acquisition of pharmacological and nonpharmacological therapies and DME. However, veterans receiving ALS care within VA clinics have limited access to clinical research. The committee believes that, given the known higher prevalence of ALS in veterans, it is critical to include the VA ALS system of care in the new integrated ALS network of care and research proposed in this report. Despite rules separating the VA system from other care systems, integration would ensure equitable and streamlined access to the highest standard of clinical care for veterans, as well as the ability to participate in clinical trials. Investment in the VA to achieve these goals would require separate, congressionally mandated funding to build a research infrastructure and organized network of care that would integrate into the proposed model of care and research recommended in this report.

Meeting the Challenge of Payment and Reimbursement for ALS Multidisciplinary Care and Research

Multidisciplinary care visits require multiple hours and involve several health professionals, but this type of care is reimbursed at the same rate as a single specialist's 30- to 60-minute office visit. This places a financial strain on ALS multidisciplinary clinics, hindering their ability to hire, retain, and expand the clinic staff to meet the needs of people living with ALS and their families. Today, larger ALS clinics rely heavily on philanthropy and institutional resources, which is unsustainable, exacerbates the significant variations in resources that exist across ALS clinics, and limits access to state-of-the-art care.

The current funding structure for ALS multidisciplinary clinics is not a sustainable model to provide high-quality care. Reimbursement policies need to promote the seamless delivery of clinical care and home-based services and equipment, including the use of telehealth to provide services across state lines—this would be similar to what VA offers veterans with ALS through their exemplary model.

The following longer-term solutions are recommended by the committee to make ALS a livable disease, with additional details about supporting evidence and proposed implementation provided in the report chapters. To develop an integrated multidisciplinary care and research system that would provide high-quality care and access to research opportunities for all people with ALS the committee offers Recommendations 4-1 through 4-4.

Recommendation 4-1: Build an inclusive and integrated ALS multidisciplinary care and research system.

The Centers for Medicare & Medicaid Services and the National Institute of Neurological Disorders and Stroke, in partnership with current ALS multidisciplinary care clinic system leaders (e.g., U.S. Department of Veterans Affairs, ALS Association, Muscular Dystrophy Association),

and community-based providers should build an inclusive and integrated multidisciplinary care and research system for people living with ALS. This network should consist of:

a. Community-Based ALS Centers,
b. Regional ALS Centers, and
c. Comprehensive ALS Care and Research Centers.

Recommendation 4-2: Improve racial and ethnic equity in the ALS care and research system.

ALS multidisciplinary clinics should partner with community members and community-serving organizations to pursue targeted approaches to understanding and improving racial and ethnic equity in ALS care and outcomes in their geographic area.

The committee believes there are several opportunities that ALS clinics, in partnership with entities that serve the local community such as Federally Qualified Health Centers, should pursue, including the following:

- Create community-focused steering committees. Each Community-Based ALS Care Center, as recommended in this report, in the newly integrated ALS care and research system should include a steering committee that would include multiple community members—individuals living with ALS, former ALS caregivers, at-risk genetic carriers, and other ALS experts from diverse racial and ethnic backgrounds, including non-English speaking individuals, among others—to build a bridge to the community and help develop programs to bring people who might otherwise go unnoticed into the ALS system.
- Collect and analyze data on racial equity. ALS centers should be expected to measure and address racial equity. Local clinics should report on the unique factors contributing to diagnostic delays in their geographic area. This responsibility to their population could be tied to funding and be a condition of qualifying as an ALS center.
- Adopt antiracism and implicit bias training as an expected and regular part of training. Each Comprehensive ALS Care and Research Center should lead antiracism and implicit bias training for center staff and clinicians that is not a one-time exercise but a regular part of training. Training would include developing an understanding of disparities in ALS, the social and structural determinants of health, and what it looks like to provide good care to diverse and historically underrepresented populations.

Recommendation 4-3: Align reimbursement to achieve the goals of the ALS clinical care and research system.

The Centers for Medicare & Medicaid Services, private insurers, the National Institutes of Health, and the National Institute of Neurological Disorders and Stroke should align reimbursement and the goals of the new, inclusive, and integrated ALS clinical care and research system.

Recommendation 4-4: Enhance access to ALS clinical care and research and education opportunities within the U.S. Department of Veterans Affairs (VA).

Congress should allocate specific funding to create a VA network for ALS clinical care, research, education, and innovation to align with the new system of care outlined in this report. VA should use these funds to resolve ALS workforce shortages, ensure access to comprehensive ALS care for veterans regardless of geographic location, increase the number of health professional training opportunities to support ALS care for veterans, and invest in clinical and informatics resources at VA to enhance existing collaboration with the Centers for Disease Control and Prevention ALS registry.

ADVANCING ALS RESEARCH AND ACCELERATING THERAPEUTIC DEVELOPMENT

The history of drug development for ALS is filled with many failures and too few successful drugs. The four unique drugs the U.S. Food and Drug Administration (FDA) has approved for ALS have limited clinical benefit.[4] Over the past decade, numerous research advances have identified a wide range of potential therapeutic pathways and potential drug targets and genes associated with ALS, but the small pool of available research participants, exacerbated by restrictive clinical trial eligibility criteria and delays from symptom onset to diagnosis and clinical trial entry, a lack of biomarkers, and overall limited understanding of the disease are factors contributing to the lack of significant success drug developers have had in the ALS realm.

The committee notes that industry, academia, the federal government, and nonprofit organizations are all involved in some manner in efforts to

---

[4] As the committee was finishing its work on this report, the company developing AMX0035/ Relyvrio announced the latest results of a Phase 3 trial in which the drug performed no better than placebo. In April 2024, the company began the process of removing Relyvrio from the market.

develop therapeutics for ALS, often in collaboration across sectors. New ALS initiatives are underway, focused primarily on enhancing funding and coordination for basic research and drug development and spurred by the 2021 Accelerating Access to Critical Therapies for ALS Act (ACT for ALS). Section 3 of ACT for ALS authorized the U.S. Department of Health and Human Services Public-Private Partnership for Rare Neurodegenerative Diseases among NIH, FDA, and other eligible entities. NIH and FDA are collaborating to establish this partnership, which has three integrated components in the design and implementation phases during this project's timeframe: (1) Critical Path for Rare Neurodegenerative Diseases (CP-RND), (2) Accelerating Medicines Partnership in ALS (AMP ALS), and (3) Access for ALL in ALS Clinical Research Consortium (ALL ALS).

Integrating Clinical Research into the ALS Care Delivery Network

Although a variety of mechanisms exist for conducting clinical trials a centralized, dedicated ALS clinical trials network that builds on and brings together existing ALS clinical trial consortia would provide a coherent approach to clinical trials and natural history studies that permits faster answers to multiple questions at once. The committee believes that a centralized, NIH-led ALS clinical trials network would provide the best of each currently available network and harmonize approaches and support to see improvement in ALS trial success.

An ALS clinical trials network would need to include participants from the entire population of individuals living with ALS, particularly individuals representing diverse ethnic and racial populations, and it should be strategic in site selection to expand the opportunities for individuals to participate who might otherwise not want to travel a long distance to participate in a clinical trial. Such a network dedicated to ALS would create an opportunity for scores of multidisciplinary ALS centers in diverse geographic areas to be designated and accredited under the new proposed nationwide integrated system of care and research to bring clinical trials closer to ALS individuals' homes across the nation.

New and Emerging Nonpharmacological Technologies

Technological advances have created opportunities for technology-mediated tools to provide support for persons with ALS and their families and improve quality of life at home. For example, advances in telehealth technology have accelerated home monitoring opportunities. Eye-tracking communication devices enable patients with advanced paralysis to communicate using eye movements. Brain–computer interfaces (BCIs) allow patients to communicate by translating brain signals into text or speech, offering an alternative communication method for those with severe motor impairments. Emerging technologies need to be developed with the engagement of end users, consideration of data privacy and security, attention to inclusive technologies that reduce rather than exacerbate health disparities and using technology to facilitate and increase access to clinical trials for individuals living with ALS.

Establishing a Comprehensive ALS Registry

A robust registry of people with ALS would help measure progress toward making ALS a more livable disease. It would collect data on care, outcomes, and risk factors, providing a valuable population-level perspective on living with ALS. Patient registries have been used to great effect in other disease spaces, such as cystic fibrosis, to collect information on patient demographics and survival while assessing clinical performance.

The Centers for Disease Control and Prevention (CDC) National ALS Registry is currently the primary nationwide effort to count ALS cases in the United States. It records demographic information for all registrants via self-enrollment or administrative data; people with ALS can provide other information, such as clinical characteristics and risk factor exposure, via optional surveys. However, the National ALS Registry is inadequate. Its data are incomplete, nonrepresentative, and not reported in a timely manner. By including registration as a routine part of care at every multidisciplinary ALS center and reporting that data more regularly, the National ALS Registry could be made more impactful as a source of population health data.

The National ALS Registry could also serve as the key population health element of a larger ALS data platform. ALS data collection today is fragmented and uncoordinated. Data are collected by natural history studies, biorepositories, state-level ALS registries, and other sources. Including ALS among CDC's list of National Notifiable Conditions would add another highly useful data source. Making the National ALS Registry interoperable with these data sources would magnify its impact and connect currently siloed data.

Recommendation 5-1: Create an ALS clinical trials network.

The National Institute of Neurological Disorders and Stroke should ensure the existence of a dedicated ALS clinical trials network distributed across diverse geographic regions in the United States, coordinated and funded by the National Institutes of Health. To be most effective, the ALS clinical trials network should be integrated with the hub-and-spoke clinical care network recommended in this report.

Recommendation 5-2: Expand ALS translational research.

The ALS-focused public–private partnerships created under the Accelerating Access for Critical Therapies for ALS Act should consider additional translational research priorities that would accelerate therapeutic developments in ALS. (See full Recommendation 5-2 in Chapter 5 for research priorities.)

Recommendation 5-3: Build a comprehensive ALS registry as part of a larger ALS data platform.

The Centers for Disease Control and Prevention (CDC) and the National Institute of Neurological Disorders and Stroke (e.g., Access for ALL in ALS Clinical Research Consortium) should integrate new and current data sources with CDC's National ALS Registry to create a comprehensive, interoperable data platform capable of collecting detailed, geocoded, longitudinal data on all individuals living with ALS, as well as people at increased genetic risk of developing ALS. To make this registry most useful, CDC and the Council of State and Territorial Epidemiologists should add ALS to the National Notifiable Diseases Surveillance System, and states should require clinicians to report all cases of ALS.

Recommendation 5-4: Fund neglected areas of research that would yield near-term gains in quality of life for people with ALS.

The National Institutes of Health, the National Institute of Neurological Disorders and Stroke, the Agency for Healthcare Research and Quality, and other ALS research funders should prioritize research to learn what works best in ALS care and increase support for other critical areas of ALS research that are currently neglected but would yield near-term gains in quality of life for persons with ALS. (Such as health services research and evaluations of nonpharmacologic interventions, services, and approaches [e.g., physical therapy, speech and language supports, and respiratory therapy]. See full Recommendation 5-4 in Chapter 5 for a list of recommended research priorities.)

PREVENTING ALS

Individuals with ALS and at-risk genetic carriers need to be able to access genetic testing and counseling. In addition to knowing valuable information about their genetic risk for developing ALS, the more people who have access to their genetic information could provide more data for researchers seeking to answer important questions about how and when

ALS develops or does not develop in certain individuals. Access to genetic testing and counseling varies widely across clinics and programs that provide reduced or no-cost genetic testing panels for ALS.

Research that identifies new targets for therapeutic intervention, biomarkers of ALS, risk factors contributing to the development of ALS, and environmental exposures that contribute to the development of ALS raises the possibility of developing agents or interventions that can delay or even prevent the development or progression of ALS. With the first prevention trial underway in an at-risk genetic carrier population (Biogen trial of tofersen) there is reason to believe additional research studies in genetic carriers will be possible in the future. To get to this point, the challenge is to develop evidence for clinical benefit and a biomarker signal in a symptomatic population before launching a study to evaluate disease progression or conversion to disease in an at-risk asymptomatic population. These studies can be long and challenging and will require increased collaboration and partnership among research funders, drug developers, and ALS nonprofit organizations and the affected communities to realize progress.

Recommendation 6-1: Increase access to genetic testing and counseling for people with ALS and their families.

Genetic testing and counseling should be made substantially more easily and consistently available for people with ALS and their families. The Centers for Medicare & Medicaid Services and private insurers should pay for genetic testing and counseling for all people living with ALS and their families. State legislatures should examine possible measures to prohibit genetic discrimination in life insurance, long-term care insurance, and disability insurance based on genetic risk for ALS.

Recommendation 6-2: Advance research focused on populations at risk of developing ALS.

Research funders should partner with drug developers and the ALS community to advance research focused on populations at risk of developing ALS, including at-risk genetic carriers. Research funders should partner with drug developers and the ALS community to develop specific research programs focused on the unique unmet needs of at-risk genetic carriers. Research funders should support large-scale, prospective natural history studies of populations at risk of ALS.

The committee finds that each of these recommendations, if implemented, would yield significant improvements in the livability of ALS today and well into the future.

1

Introduction and Study Context

Amyotrophic lateral sclerosis (ALS) is a rapidly progressive, invariably fatal neurological disease for which there are no treatments that stop or reverse disease progression. At least 30,000 individuals in the United States are estimated to have a diagnosis of ALS at any given time, though as discussed in Chapter 6, this estimate may be an undercount (Mehta et al., 2023). The pathological hallmark of ALS is progressive degeneration of motor neurons in the brain, brainstem, and spinal cord that causes a gradual loss of motor functions. As upper motor neurons in the motor cortex deteriorate, there is scarring (sclerosis) along the length of the corticospinal tract. Death of spinal cord motor neurons and resulting denervation of muscle underlie muscle wasting (amyotrophy). No two people living with ALS will experience the disease in the same way or have their disease progress at the same rate. Some people living with ALS have symptoms that progress slowly, while others progress rapidly.

Some two-thirds of individuals with ALS initially experience effects in the muscles of the hands, forearms, calves, and feet. This form of ALS is called limb-onset ALS (Wijesekera and Nigel Leigh, 2009). The other one-third of patients first experience weakness in the muscles around the mouth and throat and develop what is called bulbar-onset ALS. Over time, these symptoms progress toward other areas of the body until all muscle groups are paralyzed. As a result, people with ALS often find motor tasks such as walking, eating, and interacting with objects increasingly difficult as their disease progresses (Jellinger, 2023; Simmons, 2015), and many then require assistance with day-to-day activities. Death usually results from respiratory failure when the muscles responsible for breathing become paralyzed.

People living with ALS typically experience respiratory failure within 2 to 5 years of when symptoms first appear (Chiò et al., 2009; Wolf et al., 2014). A surgical procedure called a tracheotomy allows for artificial ventilation and breathing, and people living with ALS may undergo such a procedure to extend their lives. In doing so, people with ALS may live for many more years. For example, the famed astrophysicist Stephen Hawking lived for 55 years after his symptoms first appeared.

Despite the progression of symptoms for this always fatal disease, most people living with ALS and who are not affected by frontotemporal dementia (FTD) retain cognitive function. However, ALS can also present with symptoms of cognitive impairment more frequently than in patients with other neuromuscular diseases (Ferrari et al., 2011; Jellinger, 2023).

When cognitive impairment does occur in people with ALS, it is frequently associated with behavioral dysfunction similar to cognitive impairment observed in people with FTD (Ferrari et al., 2011). The spectrum of cognitive and behavioral dysfunction in persons with ALS is broad, ranging from mild cognitive decline to clinically confirmed FTD (Jellinger, 2023). FTD can cause dramatic behavior or personality changes, socially inappropriate or repetitive behaviors, agitation, and an inability to use language.

The reported frequency of cognitive impairment in persons with ALS varies greatly between 30 percent to 75 percent, with up to 45 percent of persons with ALS exhibiting clinically confirmed FTD (Jellinger, 2023). The cognitive and behavioral changes come with shared pathological and genetic features of these two diseases, which are often called the disease continuum or spectrum disease of ALS and FTD.

The symptoms of ALS progress over the natural history of the disease. While these are widely recognized as hallmarks of ALS, ALS is a multisystem disease with a high prevalence of secondary symptoms including fatigue, pain, insomnia, anxiety, depression, and dyspnea (Brizzi et al., 2020; Jaafar et al., 2021; Nicholson et al., 2018). The impact of secondary symptoms affecting quality of life is not as well recognized. For example, while ALS was once described as a disease characterized by "painless weakness," it is now known that pain is a common secondary symptom affecting persons with ALS (Goutman, 2017). Most pain experienced by people with ALS is caused by tissue damage, although they can also experience other pain subtypes, such as pain caused by nerve damage (Chiò et al., 2017). Shoulder pain is a common example of pain affecting people with ALS, with an estimated prevalence of 23 percent in one population-based retrospective study involving 193 patients (Ho et al., 2011).

EPIDEMIOLOGY

ALS incidence increases with age and peaks around 60 to 79 years. Since there are approximately 30,000 people living with ALS, it is considered a rare disease, which the Orphan Drug Act of 1992 defines as a disease or condition affecting fewer than 200,000 people in the United States (FDA, 2013). Although ALS is technically a rare disease, the lethality of the disease and the short lifespan greatly reduce the number of individuals alive with ALS at any one time. The number of new cases each year in the United States is approximately 5,000, compared to approximately 360 new cases of Duchenne muscular dystrophy and 10,000 new cases of multiple sclerosis annually. The number of people expected to develop the disease around the world in any given year is an estimated 1.68 per 100,000, though this varies slightly by region (Longinetti and Fang, 2019; Marin et al., 2017; Xu et al., 2020) and sex (Fontana et al., 2021). The number of new cases of ALS is expected to rise in the future (Arthur et al., 2016; Gowland et al., 2019). This is a result of demographic changes, such as the aging of the population and an increase in exposure to potential environmental risk factors.

The Centers for Disease Control and Prevention (CDC) National ALS Registry data report a prevalence of 9.1 per 100,000 in 2018 (Mehta et al., 2023) in the United States, though as discussed in Chapter 6, this may be a significant undercount. ALS global crude prevalence is 4.42 per 100,000 but varies slightly by region and sex (Xu, 2020). The data from only a few countries are reliable, but the available data can show patterns and useful information about the prevalence of ALS outside of the United States (Blank et al., 2021). The highest prevalence of ALS is found in Australia (8.7), Belgium (8–12), Canada (8.1), Ireland (8), Italy (10.5), Japan (7–8), Nigeria (15), and the United Kingdom (7) (all per 100,000). The lowest prevalence of ALS can be found in China (1.23), India (4), Mexico (1.44), Pakistan (1.44), Russia (0.7–1.25), South Korea (3.43), and Tunisia (0.45) (all per 100,000) (Blank et al., 2021).

STUDY TASK

In response to the devastating nature of ALS for individuals and their families, Congress, as noted in the Consolidated Appropriations Act of 2022,[1] directed the National Institutes of Health (NIH) to commission a study by the National Academies of Sciences, Engineering, and Medicine (the National Academies) to identify and recommend actions for the public, private, and nonprofit sectors to undertake that would make ALS a livable disease within a decade. The National Institute of Neurological Disorders and Stroke (NINDS) contracted with the National Academies to address the statement of task (see Box 1-1).

---

[1] See House Report 117-96, originally accompanying Labor, Health and Human Services, Education, Agriculture, Rural Development, Energy and Water Development, Financial Services and General Government, Interior, Environment, Military Construction, Veterans Affairs, Transportation, and Housing and Urban Development Appropriations Act, 2022, H.R. 4502, as consolidated in Consolidated Appropriations Act of 2022, Public Law 117-103, 117th Congress (March 15, 2022).

BOX 1-1
Statement of Task

An ad hoc committee of the National Academies of Sciences, Engineering, and Medicine will conduct a study to identify and recommend key actions for the public, private, and nonprofit sectors to undertake to make amyotrophic lateral sclerosis (ALS) a livable disease within a decade. The committee will consider the landscape of ALS therapeutic development, care, services, and supports, such as:

- pathways for developing more effective and meaningful treatments and a cure;
- interventions to reduce and prevent the progression and complications of ALS;
- challenges and obstacles for public, private, and nonprofit sectors to overcome to make ALS a livable disease within a decade;
- the type and range of care and services people with ALS and their families need and how to ensure they receive comprehensive, quality care;
- what care, services, and preventive measures people at-risk of ALS need; and
- how to improve the quality of life, health, and well-being of affected individuals and families.

The committee's work will consider equity issues across the landscape and build on priorities identified in the National Institute of Neurological Disorders and Stroke's ALS Strategic Plan, the U.S. Food and Drug Administration's Action Plan for Rare Neurodegenerative Diseases including ALS, and additional existing analyses and expert and public input. The committee will develop a report with its recommendations for key actions that federal agencies, the pharmaceutical industry, and non-governmental organizations can take, including identifying opportunities for collaboration.

THE NATURE OF ALS AND ITS SYMPTOMS

As discussed earlier, ALS is a neurodegenerative disease most commonly characterized by symptoms such as difficulty walking, breathing, and speaking; weakness in hands and limbs; and muscle twitching. Chapter 2 discusses these and other symptoms through the lens of care and management. However, the course of ALS is variable; no two people with ALS will experience the disease the same way. Exposure to risk factors, age of onset, clinical phenotype, and developmental course all differ from person to person.

Risk Factors of ALS

There are two main types of ALS. Sporadic ALS is the most common form, accounting for approximately 90 percent of all cases and occurs randomly in individuals without a family history of ALS. However, approximately 10 to 15 percent of individuals with sporadic ALS have mutations in genes known to be associated with ALS cases (Chia et al., 2018; Goutman et al., 2022d). The term *familial ALS* refers to individuals with ALS who have a family history of the disease. Of those individuals with familial ALS, 70 percent are carriers of known gene mutations associated with ALS.

Identifying risk factors for ALS has been a key component of research into the disease. It allows people to better assess their personal risk of ALS. Knowledge about the genetic components of ALS may help inform models of the disease's development, while identifying environmental risk factors may help reduce risk by reducing exposure. Further discussion of ALS prevention can be found in Chapter 6. However, research into gene–environment interactions into ALS remains nascent, and further investigation is warranted.

Genetic Risk Factors

Genetics are thought to be a large component of risk in ALS, affecting both familial ALS and sporadic ALS. The most prevalent gene mutations related to ALS risk include C9orf72, SOD1, TDP-43, and FUS (Chia et al., 2018). However, research has identified close to 50 genes associated with ALS when mutated, with additional gene variants that are considered risk factors of ALS disease manifestation. Mutations can be either monogenic (occurring in one gene) or polygenic (occurring in many), though research into polygenic risk is ongoing (Dou et al., 2023). These gene variations often lead to a loss of function of the affected gene, which disrupts normal cellular processes and produces the physiological phenomena associated with ALS, such as neuronal or glial dysfunction.

Known ALS genetic mutations vary in their frequency, penetrance, inheritance pattern, and associated phenotypes and pathology. Frequency refers to how common the mutation is in ALS populations, which can be further disaggregated by familial/sporadic ALS, race or ethnicity, and other demographic factors.

Penetrance is how likely a carrier (i.e., someone with the gene) is to develop the disease. Higher penetrance means many carriers develop disease, while lower penetrance means fewer carriers develop disease. Carriers who have yet to develop ALS are a genetically defined population of interest in many studies, especially those examining preventive strategies (Benatar et al., 2022a). Penetrance varies by ALS genetic mutation, and mutations to the most common, such as C9orf72 and SOD1, are often highly penetrant (Goutman et al., 2022d). Importantly, some genes related to ALS do not definitively cause the disease but instead confer risk. Some evidence further suggests that penetrance of a genetic mutation may be related to other environmental exposures (Westeneng et al., 2021).

Heritability for genetic mutations related to ALS varies. These genes are typically autosomal dominant, meaning that only a single copy of the mutation on a nonsex chromosome is sufficient to cause disease or modify risk. However, recessive inheritance, which requires inheritance of two mutated copies, occurs for some genes, as does sex-linked inheritance. Estimates of heritability in ALS-associated genes have ranged from 8.5 percent to 61 percent (Al-Chalabi et al., 2010; van Rheenen et al., 2016).

ALS genes also impact onset age, phenotype, development of cognitive or behavioral involvement, rate of disease progression, and survival (Goutman et al., 2022d). For instance, mutations in the C9orf72 gene are strongly associated with the co-development of FTD. In many instances, the specific mutation to the ALS gene impacts all these characteristics (McCann et al., 2017). For example, a variant of the SOD1 gene with what is called the A5V mutation is very rapidly progressive. However, the full spectrum of genotype-phenotype relations in ALS remains incompletely known, particularly since new ALS genes and variants continue to be discovered.

Environmental Risk Factors

Research has linked contributions from environmental exposures to the development of sporadic ALS (Al-Chalabi and Hardiman, 2013; Chiò et al., 2018). The ALS "exposome" refers to the sum of environmental exposures and lifestyle habits that contribute to ALS risk (Goutman et al., 2023). Identifying environmental risk factors may allow for disease prevention in several ways. For example, exposure to known risk factors can be eliminated. When exposure cannot be fully eliminated, such as when it is related to home or occupational factors, it may still be possible to mitigate risk of ALS onset. Polluted areas could be cleaned up, and employees could use personal protective equipment when necessary. Finally, based on their genetic and environmental exposures, genetic carriers may benefit from prophylactic gene therapies currently being tested (Benatar et al., 2022b).

Systematic reviews and meta-analyses have suggested multiple environmental risks (Newell et al., 2022; Wang et al., 2017). These include:

- pesticides (Andrew et al., 2021a; Goutman et al., 2019; Su et al., 2016);
- metals (Andrew et al., 2018; Figueroa-Romero et al., 2020; Peters et al., 2021);
- air pollution (Myung et al., 2019; Nunez et al., 2022; Parks et al., 2022; Seelen et al., 2017);
- electromagnetic exposure (Koeman et al., 2017; Luna et al., 2019; Peters et al., 2019);

- one's microbiome (Boddy et al., 2021; Di Gioia et al., 2020; Hertzberg et al., 2022; Nicholson et al., 2021);
- being a veteran, particularly when exposed to environmental toxicants or trauma (Cragg et al., 2017; McKay et al., 2021; Sagiraju et al., 2020);
- working in certain occupations likely to encounter toxic environmental exposures (Goutman et al., 2022b), such as:
  - production (Goutman et al., 2022a);
  - agriculture (Filippini et al., 2020b);
  - mechanics (Andrew et al., 2017, 2021b);
  - painting (Andrew et al., 2017, 2021b);
  - construction (Andrew et al., 2017, 2021b); and
  - glass, pottery, and tile work (Peters et al., 2017).
- exposure to repeated physical trauma (Andrew et al., 2021b; Filippini et al., 2020a; Pupillo et al., 2018); and
- other variables (e.g., socioeconomic status, education, exercise, alcohol, smoking) (Goutman et al., 2022c; Henry et al., 2015; Peters et al., 2020; Westeneng et al., 2021).

Investigators do not consider the link between these and the development of sporadic ALS to be conclusive, and genetic status may modify environmental risk (Westeneng et al., 2021). Concordance is not 100 percent across studies, and further investigation is needed to determine the role of genetics in modifying environmental risk.

Age

Age is one of the strongest known risk factors for ALS. Older onset age is more common, but, nevertheless, like presentation, is variable. Juvenile (<25 years of age) and young-onset (<45 years of age) ALS are possible (Souza et al., 2024; Turner et al., 2012). Studies suggest that onset age varies with ALS subtype (see Table 1-1) as well as genetic mutation. Older onset age results in an older peak prevalence. In the United States, the National ALS Registry reports peak ALS prevalence between 60 to 79 years (Feldman et al., 2022).

Development of ALS

Pre-Symptomatic Phase

Prior to disease onset, individuals are susceptible to ALS either by harboring pathogenic mutations to ALS genes, by various risk-enhancing exposures, or through combined gene-exposure interactions (Benatar et al., 2022b; Goutman et al., 2023). Preventative strategies may be feasible during this phase, but research is still ongoing (Benatar et al., 2023). People with ALS

TABLE 1-1 ALS Subtypes, Mean Onset Age, Median Survival, and Other Characteristics

ALS Subtype	Approx. Percentage of Cases	Mean Onset Age	Mean Diagnostic Delay	Male to Female Incidence	Median Survival	Approx. Proportion Frontotemporal Dementia
Spinal onset	30.3%	62.8 years	10.9 months	1.65:1	2.6 years	4%
Bulbar onset	34.2%	68.8 years	9.8 months	0.98:1	2.0 years	9%
Flail leg	13.0%	65.0 years	13.1 months	1.03:1	3.0 years	4.1%
Flail arm	5.5%	62.6 years	12.8 months	4.00:1	4.0 years	1.4%
Pyramidal	9.1%	58.3 years	15.9 months	1.04:1	6.3 years	2.5%
Primary lateral sclerosis	4.0%	58.9 years	15.9 months	0.98:1	13.1 years	3.8%
Progressive muscular atrophy	2.9%	56.2 years	15.5 months	2.04:1	7.3 years	0%
Respiratory onset	1.1%	65.2 years	6.4 months	6.00:1	1.4 years	0%

NOTE: Data are broadly representative and specific characteristics vary by ALS population.
SOURCE: Generated by the committee with data from Chiò et al., 2011.

first experience a pre-symptomatic phase lacking overt symptoms. This phase is further broken down into an earlier, clinically silent "pre-manifest" phase and a "prodromal" phase characterized by early symptoms. Some sensitive biomarker tests may detect evidence of the disease during the pre-manifest phase, although there is no clinically approved test. Blood or cerebrospinal fluid levels of a protein called neurofilament light chain, a marker of neuronal injury, may be promising (Benatar et al., 2018). During the prodromal phase, patients exhibit signs and symptoms not meeting the formal diagnostic criteria for ALS, such as mild motor, mild cognitive, and mild behavioral impairments, which may go unnoticed.

Presentation and Subtypes of ALS

Eventually, people with pre-symptomatic ALS enter a clinically manifest phase where diagnosis becomes possible, with subsequent disease progression until death. This presentation is highly variable with several clinical subtypes (Feldman et al., 2022; Goutman et al., 2022e). One variable is the onset segment, meaning the part of the spinal cord and the corresponding muscles that are first affected by the disease (see Figure 1-1, Part B). A second variable is motor neuron involvement; ALS presentation can involve lower and/or upper motor neurons (see Figure 1-1, Part A).

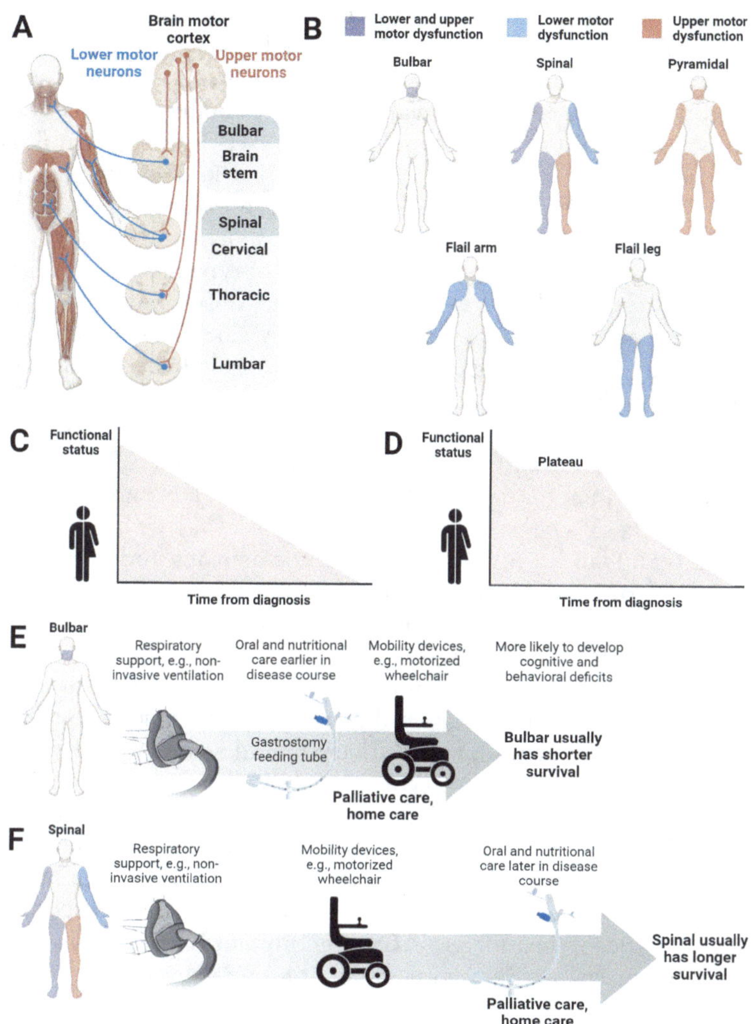

FIGURE 1-1 Most common ALS subtypes, natural history, and multidisciplinary treatment.

NOTES: (A) Lower (blue) and upper (red) motor neurons and spinal segments and corresponding areas initially affected by bulbar versus spinal onset ALS. (B) ALS subtypes and lower and/or upper motor neuron involvement in color legend. ALS progression is variable and can be relatively constant (C) versus punctuated by plateau periods without progression (D). Treatment will differ for (E) bulbar versus (F) spinal onset ALS. For instance, bulbar ALS patients may require oral and nutritional care earlier in their disease course than spinal onset ALS patients. Conversely, spinal onset ALS patients may require mobility assistance earlier in their disease course than bulbar onset patients. SOURCE: Adapted from Feldman et al., 2022.

Lower motor neurons connect the muscles to the spinal cord whereas upper motor neurons connect the spinal cord to the brain.

"Spinal" and "bulbar" ALS are the two most common subtypes. Although the precise percentage varies across populations, generally, they each constitute about one-third of ALS cases (see Table 1-1). Bulbar ALS involves both upper and lower motor neurons and affects facial muscles; this often presents as difficulty speaking and/or swallowing. Spinal ALS involves both upper and lower motor neurons and causes muscle weakness in limbs. The cervical-onset spinal subtype first affects the arms, especially by causing hand weakness; lumbar-onset spinal subtype first impacts the legs, especially by causing foot weakness. However, muscle weakness eventually spreads to all limbs and spinal segments, including respiratory muscles.

Besides spinal and bulbar ALS, the remaining third of cases present as flail leg (approx. 13% of total ALS), flail arm (approx. 5.5%), pyramidal (approx. 9%), primary lateral sclerosis (approx. 4%), progressive muscular atrophy (approx. 3%), respiratory onset (approx. 1%), or hemiplegic (rare) (see Table 1-1). Flail leg involves lower motor neurons and affects the legs, whereas flail arm instead affects the arms but also predominantly affects lower motor neuron (although progressive disease impacts some upper motor neurons). Primary lateral sclerosis is an upper motor neuron manifestation impacting limb and facial muscles, while progressive muscular atrophy affects the same muscles as well as respiratory muscles but manifests with lower motor neuron injury. Primary lateral sclerosis and progressive muscular atrophy are sometimes considered distinct entities from ALS, but many ALS neurologists consider them to be part of the same disease spectrum as ALS. Pyramidal ALS is like primary lateral sclerosis but eventually involves lower motor neurons. Respiratory onset ALS impacts both upper and lower motor neurons and initiates in the respiratory muscles. Finally, the rare subtype of hemiplegic ALS predominantly affects upper motor neurons but causes muscle weakness only on one side of the body.

ALS Natural History and Survival

Like phenotypic presentation, the progression rate of ALS and overall survival from the time of diagnosis is highly variable. Death from ALS typically occurs due to respiratory failure and generally occurs within 2 to 5 years from diagnosis (Feldman et al., 2022; Goutman et al., 2022e). However, about 10 to 20 percent of ALS patients survive longer than 10 years; this is typically seen in people with younger-onset ALS (Chiò et al., 2009). ALS subtype affects survival (see Table 1-1), as do genetics and cognitive involvement (Chiò et al., 2009; Feldman et al., 2022; Goutman et al., 2022d; McCann et al., 2017). Increasingly, environmental factors are also being identified as influential on survival; factors investigated include exposure to persistent organic pollutants and holding occupations with hazardous occupational exposures, such as manufacturing occupations or occupational pesticides exposure (Goutman et al., 2019, 2024).

ALS progression is assessed by the Revised ALS Functional Rating Score (ALSFRS-R). Staging systems have also been developed to describe the stage of disease, the further along in stage the shorter the remaining survival time (Feldman et al., 2022; Goutman et al., 2022d). Progression is not always linear, and the disease course can be punctuated with periods without progression called "plateaus" (see Figure 1-1, Parts C and D). A population-based study of 1,214 ALS cases suggests that about one out of six people with ALS experiences a plateau lasting at least 6 months, but some experience plateaus as long as 12 or 18 months (Vasta et al., 2020). In the study population, plateaus usually occurred earlier in the disease course and were more frequent in spinal onset ALS.

There is no prognostic model in clinical practice to predict overall survival. However, the European Network for the Cure of Amyotrophic Lateral Sclerosis generated a personalized algorithm based on onset age, time to diagnosis, clinical progression rate, respiratory function, bulbar onset, confidence in the ALS diagnosis, cognitive involvement, and presence of C9orf72 mutations (Westeneng et al., 2018).

Diagnosing ALS

By the time symptoms become sufficiently evident for a clinical diagnosis of ALS, the disease has already progressed at the molecular and cellular level, and motor neuron injury is already present. Even upon symptom onset, it sometimes takes 10 to 16 months to definitively diagnose an individual with ALS, although some subtypes with a more distinct presentation, such as respiratory and bulbar onset, have shorter times to a diagnosis (Richards et al., 2021) (see Table 1-1).

There are several reasons for this diagnostic delay. First, ALS is a rare disease, so it may not occur to a general physician that they are presented with a case, which may delay referral to a specialist. However, a few core clinical factors and symptoms may prompt consideration of ALS, including family history of ALS or other neurodegenerative diseases, progressive difficulty talking or eating, limb weakness without sensory symptoms, unexplained weight loss, pseudobulbar affect, and cognitive or behavioral changes (Feldman et al., 2022). Conversely, predominantly sensory or autonomic, nonprogressive, or no-weakness manifestations should preclude ALS. The ALS Association launched the thinkALS tool to promote consideration of ALS based on core clinical and symptom presentations (ALS Association, 2021).

Second, even once a person with ALS has been referred to a specialist, the illness can mimic other conditions, so other more common causes must be ruled out before definitively diagnosing ALS. This is especially critical, since some conditions that mimic ALS are treatable. Nevertheless, due to its similar presentation and symptoms to other illnesses, ALS can be initially misdiagnosed. This may cause a person with ALS to incur unnecessary tests or cause them to miss tests that would have otherwise facilitated a more rapid diagnosis. A misdiagnosis also takes a significant emotional toll on an individual if the diagnosis is revised from a treatable condition to a terminal one, such as ALS.

An accurate, timely, and earlier ALS diagnosis is the optimal scenario, since there is evidence to suggest that earlier treatment can improve outcomes. A large analysis of 4,778 ALS patients found that delaying riluzole initiation by 1 year may shorten median survival from disease onset by 1.9 months (Thakore et al., 2022). Evidence also suggests that multidisciplinary care may improve outcomes for people with ALS across multiple domains (Miller et al., 2009). Furthermore, an earlier diagnosis would also offer ALS patients more time to contemplate and seek opportunities for clinical trial enrollment. It may also affect clinical trial eligibility. Eligibility criteria for many ALS trials exclude participants with more advanced disease in order to evaluate effectiveness before molecular and cellular development of the disease. Finally, given the typical post-diagnosis survival of only 2 to 5 years, an earlier diagnosis would give people with ALS and their families more time to plan their future financial, legal, social, psychological, and spiritual well-being.

Currently, ALS diagnosis continues to incur delays. Faster ALS diagnosis may be facilitated by encouraging earlier consideration of ALS, such as with thinkALS. For future approaches, better coordination between primary care centers and multidisciplinary ALS care centers could streamline referrals. Development of sensitive biomarker tests, especially for people exposed to genetic or environmental risk factors for ALS, might also help diagnosis of people with ALS in the pre-manifest phase.

Treating ALS

Individuals with ALS lack effective disease-modifying therapies. There are only two FDA-approved therapies that may marginally influence or alter the disease course. Riluzole, an antiglutamate agent, slows progression and increases survival by a few months. Edaravone, an antioxidant, is of uncertain efficacy and not been definitively established as broadly helpful for all people with ALS (Goutman et al., 2022d). The cornerstone of ALS care beyond these two therapies is multidisciplinary care, which is a comprehensive plan to manage symptoms in ALS patients, including respiratory and oral symptoms; nutrition and gastrointestinal symptoms; pain and symptoms secondary to muscle loss; and cognition, behavioral, and mood changes (Miller et al., 2009).

Overall, ALS treatments must be dynamic and proactive as interventions that are useful early in the disease may be different than what is useful later. Multidisciplinary care contributes to making ALS a livable condition by alleviating symptoms, helping procure equipment, and helping the individual with ALS maintain some function to navigate their day-to-day life. For instance, a motorized wheelchair can provide an individual with ALS increased movement and independence. Multidisciplinary care also supports the caregiver when the medical equipment needed to facilitate care is available. For example, an eye tracker or laser pointer can help an individual with ALS communicate with their caregiver.

Timing of multidisciplinary care services will depend on the ALS subtype. For instance, feeding tube insertion often occurs earlier in individuals with bulbar onset ALS, since facial muscles are the first to weaken. Another treatment element varying significantly across ALS cases is whether the individual suffers from cognitive and behavioral deficits. This has important implications for caregiving support and for the individual with ALS, who needs to make end-of-life decisions earlier in their disease course before cognitive impairment becomes too severe.

Since ALS is a terminal illness, people with ALS will require palliative care in addition to supportive care, especially with progressive disease. Importantly, initiation of palliative care needs to be early in the disease course to ensure continued quality of life for individuals with ALS. Although palliative care in ALS can be delivered by a multidisciplinary team, it may need to be coordinated with local providers as individuals with ALS become less able to travel.

STUDY APPROACH AND SCOPE

The National Academies Study Process

The National Academies established a committee of 18 volunteer experts with the experience and skills to accomplish the statement of task.[2] The committee included individuals with expertise in these areas: neurology, rehabilitation, pulmonary and primary care; translational ALS and FTD research; health law and policy; ethics; health care financing; nursing and long-term care; and therapeutic development and regulatory pathways,

---

[2] See https://www.nationalacademies.org/about for a detailed overview of the National Academies and see https://www.nationalacademies.org/about/our-study-process for an overview of the National Academies' study process (accessed June 10, 2024).

as well individuals with ALS lived experience. The committee convened for three in-person meetings, five virtual meetings, three virtual public workshops, and numerous committee subgroup meetings during which they gathered information, reviewed evidence, and discussed findings, conclusions, and recommendations.[3] The committee's public workshops are summarized in a Proceedings of a Workshop—in Brief, released publicly in November 2023 (NASEM, 2023).

Study Context Within the ALS Ecosystem and Related ALS Activities and Initiatives

This National Academies study ran in parallel with the launch or implementation of a broad range of new ALS initiatives focused primarily on enhancing funding and coordination for basic research and drug development, spurred by the 2021 Accelerating Access to Critical Therapies for ALS Act (ACT for ALS). These initiatives were mounted by a diverse range of groups, including NINDS, the U.S. Food and Drug Administration (FDA), and public–private partnerships such as the Critical Path for Rare Neurodegenerative Diseases. ACT for ALS initiatives primarily support expanded access to investigational therapies and accelerated development of therapeutic interventions for ALS. The committee developing this National Academies report was cognizant of these other parallel activities and its recommendations are intended to complement them.

In fiscal year (FY) 2023, NIH spent $219 million on ALS research (NIH, 2024). NIH funds a broad portfolio of ALS research including: identifying the genetic and environmental contributions to both sporadic and familial ALS; characterizing cellular processes that cause motor neuron degeneration and may be targets for intervention; understanding disease heterogeneity and progression; developing new research tools and resources; discovering biomarkers for facilitating diagnosis or clinical trials; and optimizing current therapies and developing new therapies to slow, stop, or prevent ALS or to restore communication, mobility, and independence.

Investigator-initiated research forms the foundation of NIH's ALS research portfolio, but NIH also supports several large programs for ALS research, such as the Accelerating Leading-edge Science in ALS initiative, which supports multidisciplinary team science to advance our understanding of what triggers ALS and what drives the rapid progression of this disease, and The CReATe Consortium (The Clinical Research in ALS and

---

[3]Information on the study process, committee meetings, and recordings of public sessions is available on the project webpage: https://www.nationalacademies.org/our-work/amyotrophic-lateral-sclerosis-accelerating-treatments-and-improving-quality-of-life (accessed June 10, 2024).

Related Disorders for Therapeutic Development), part of the trans-NIH Rare Diseases Clinical Research Network, which aims to accelerate the development of effective treatments by characterizing disease heterogeneity, improving existing clinical outcome measures for early- to mid-phase clinical trials, validating biomarkers as "fit for purpose," and reducing barriers for patient participation in clinical research.

Passage of ACT for ALS in 2021 and subsequent annual appropriations to NIH for implementing the ACT for ALS enabled the establishment of large clinical research programs for ALS.

Section 2 of ACT for ALS authorized the expanded access research grant program to conduct scientific research and to provide access to investigational therapies to people not otherwise eligible for clinical trials. The program is open to phase 3 or phase 2/3 clinical trial sites for investigational drugs or biological products sponsored by a small business concern (HHS, 2023).

Section 3 of ACT for ALS authorized the HHS Public-Private Partnership for Rare Neurodegenerative Diseases among NIH, FDA, and other eligible entities. NIH and FDA are collaborating to establish this partnership, which has three integrated components in the design and implementation phases during this project's timeframe: (1) Critical Path for Rare Neurodegenerative Diseases (CP-RND), (2) Accelerating Medicines Partnership in ALS (AMP ALS), and (3) Access for ALL in ALS Clinical Research Consortium (ALL ALS). Specific research activities within the public–private partnership are being guided by the NIH ALS Strategic Research Priorities, which were developed by the ALS community, including researchers, clinicians, advocates, and people with lived experience of ALS, to create a roadmap for research that will lead to effective therapies, prevention strategies, and improved quality of life (NIH, 2023). Developed by the ALS community, including researchers, clinicians, advocates, and people with lived experience of ALS, the priorities create a research roadmap for the ALS community and are being used by NIH to guide current and future investments.

Congress appropriated $25 million in FY 2022,[4] and $75 million in FYs 2023[5] and 2024[6] to NIH for implementing ACT for ALS. These funds are required to first be used to fund all expanded access research grants deemed meritorious by NIH peer review. If any funds remain, they are to be used to support the public–private partnership.

---

[4]Public Law 117-103.
[5]Public Law 117-328.
[6]Public Law 118-47.

Critical Path for Rare Neurodegenerative Diseases (CP-RND)

In September 2022 NIH and FDA announced that the Critical Path Institute (C-Path) was selected to establish a public–private partnership involving FDA, NIH, persons with lived experience, advocates, researchers, and industry to advance research in ALS and other rare neurodegenerative diseases (FDA, 2024). The CP-RND efforts will focus on landscaping activities to inform research projects supported through the initiative, generation of standards, and creation of drug development tools such as biomarkers, digital health technologies, trial simulation tools, biological disease classification, and novel clinical outcome assessments to accelerate ALS clinical trials (C-Path, n.d.).

Accelerating Medicines Partnership in ALS (AMP ALS)

The Accelerated Medicines Partnership (AMP) program through the Foundation for the National Institutes of Health (FNIH) consists of partnerships between public- and private-sector partners intended to transform the current model for developing new diagnostics and treatments (FNIH, 2023). AMP ALS was convened by FNIH and is guided by input from people with ALS lived experience. During the project's design phase, which was launched in June 2023, the steering committee was co-chaired by Dan Doctoroff, Target ALS; Stephanie Fradette, Biogen; and Amelie Gubitz, NINDS. Participants in the design phase included nine pharmaceutical companies, eight nonprofit organizations, federal partners (NIH, FDA), people with ALS lived experience, as well as FNIH and C-Path (ex officio). Following conclusion of the design phase, the AMP ALS implementation phase was launched in May 2024.

AMP ALS has the goal of establishing a comprehensive strategy to expedite the development of effective new ALS treatments and seeks to achieve this goal through (1) establishing a central ALS Knowledge Platform for data sharing and analysis; (2) developing validated biomarkers for early diagnosis and treatment assessment; (3) improving clinical outcome assessments; and (4) discovering new therapeutic targets and risk factors (FNIH, 2024). The AMP ALS partners, in consultation with people with ALS lived experience, will direct research studies to achieve these objectives through the analysis of both existing and prospectively collected longitudinal clinical and biologic datasets as well as biospecimens collected from people living with ALS or at high risk of developing ALS. Key deliverables from AMP ALS include:

- ALS Knowledge Platform—large-scale harmonized, longitudinal ALS clinical and molecular datasets comprising all stages of ALS, including pre-symptomatic familial ALS. The ALS Knowledge Platform will be a one-stop shop for academic and industry researchers to access high-value, deidentified clinical and molecular data.

- Multimodal molecular analyses of longitudinal biofluid samples and post-mortem tissue, including whole genome, gene expression, targeted and untargeted proteomics data.
- New biofluid-based and digital biomarkers to aid in early diagnosis, monitor disease progression, as well as response to treatment.
- New clinical outcome assessments, including patient-informed clinical outcome assessments (C-Path, 2024).

Access for All in ALS Clinical Research Consortium (ALL ALS)

In October 2023, NINDS announced initial awards for ALL ALS (NINDS, 2023a). The consortium will provide a large, scalable clinical research infrastructure with the goal of facilitating research aimed at obtaining mechanistic insights into ALS heterogeneity and identifying therapeutic targets and biomarkers (NINDS, 2023b). ALL ALS will undertake a comprehensive longitudinal natural history study, collecting a wealth of longitudinal clinical data and associated biospecimens that will be shared through the ALS Knowledge Platform and established NIH biorepositories, respectively. The planned natural history study will include individuals with symptomatic ALS, asymptomatic gene carriers, and controls. To increase outreach to potential participants, the consortium will develop community engagement strategies to reach a broad population of people living with ALS or at high risk for developing ALS, and deploy decentralized clinical research methodologies to allow individuals to remotely enroll and be monitored in research studies. The AMP ALS steering committee and NIH will guide the implementation of ALL ALS. An AMP ALS working group will closely collaborate with ALL ALS to provide input on the various study protocols.

Collaboration

The initiatives described above are each applying their unique lens to the work and their collaboration, as well as to the ALL ALS network, to identify the best opportunities to develop effective drug development tools. The ALL ALS consortium will be the space where the drug development tools and approaches developed by CP-RND and AMP ALS will be tested and refined. At the time of this report's writing, each initiative was just getting underway and moving beyond the design phase. To highlight one piece of work, as part of the landscaping effort to identify unmet needs, CP-RND reviewed more than 70 ALS datasets in the United States and around the world, including information on the data collected and the architecture of the data system. CP-RND is in progress to finalize 18 agreements that would allow the extraction and curation of datasets. Sharing this information with

AMP ALS, the goal is to ensure that the creation of any new data infrastructure is appropriately building on what has been done and is truly addressing an unmet need (C-Path, 2024). In early 2024, CP-RND and AMP ALS began the process of bringing in datasets from a variety of industry and other databases for harmonization into an ALS Knowledge Platform, which will be broadly accessible for research purposes. Another ongoing effort of CP-RND is to evaluate opportunities to improve the ALSFRS (the widely used tool for measuring ALS disease progression) to measure outcomes that are most meaningful to persons with ALS.

Centering on ALS Lived Experiences

The committee centered this study around the lived experience of those affected by ALS. This includes people living with ALS, caregivers, and at-risk genetic carriers, and the committee included several people with such perspectives on its roster. In addition, members of the ALS community and others shared public comments with the committee during public workshops and via a public email address. The committee also received feedback from six consultants with lived experience who responded to some of the committee's draft report text and recommendations to consider their relevance to the ALS community. Box 1-2 lists these lived experience consultants. The lived experience of ALS is discussed throughout this report, particularly in Chapter 2, and the committee based much of its analysis on the perspectives that people living with ALS provided. The contributions of the committee members with lived experience, speakers, and consultants, as well as the ALS community, were invaluable to this study.

Overarching Goals of the Report

The primary goal of this report in the short term is to ensure that all individuals suffering from ALS have access to affordable, state-of-the art multidisciplinary treatment and services. The longer-term goal is, as specified in the committee's statement of task, to make ALS a livable disease in 10 years. What that means is laid out in more detail in Chapter 2 but, in summary, it means to significantly increase both survivability and quality of life for everyone affected by this disease, including people living with ALS, people at genetic risk of developing ALS, and their families and caregivers.

Despite the heroic efforts undertaken at ALS clinics every day across the country, many people living with ALS experience significant delays in diagnosis and never receive the multidisciplinary care they need. Black individuals with ALS experience a 50 percent longer delay in receiving an ALS diagnosis even though Black individuals living with ALS, in one study, were found to live closer to a multidisciplinary ALS center than White people

BOX 1-2
Lived Experience Consultants

The National Academies and the committee thank these individuals, who served as volunteer lived experience consultants, for sharing their perspectives with the committee. The consultants reviewed select portions of the committee's draft report text and recommendations.

Michael Cosgray is a presymptomatic genetic carrier of the C9orf72 mutation that can cause ALS. Michael lost multiple family members to ALS and saw the impact of the disease on his mother, who was a fast progressor and died on April 11, 2004. Michael made the decision early in life not to have children to avoid the risk of passing down this devastating mutation to future generations.

Desiree Galvez Kessler was diagnosed with ALS at age 28 shortly after giving birth to her daughter. Desi is a volunteer member of a support organization, Her ALS Story. The group seeks to raise awareness of the impact ALS has on young women diagnosed before age 35 and provide a community for them to connect, learn from each other, and find support so they can live their best lives.

Bernadine A. Okeke was diagnosed with ALS in 2019 at age 63. She is a volunteer member of the Many Shades of ALS Community Team at I AM ALS, a nonprofit advocacy organization. The Community Team brings attention to, and provides resources for, the mental, physical, and social health of people of color living with and affected by ALS.

Ann Oliff is a caregiver for her spouse, Layne Oliff, who was diagnosed with primary lateral sclerosis in 2017 and then ALS in 2020 after lower motor neuron symptoms emerged. Ann retired from her career as a nurse and massage therapist to provide full-time care for Layne. She previously served on a pharmaceutical company patient advisory board related to her experience as an ALS caregiver.

Kristin Rankin was diagnosed with ALS at age 38. She is a supportive mom to three daughters—ages 15, 12, and 10—who provide inspiration to live life to the fullest and remain hopeful. Since 2022, she has served as a volunteer with the Community Outreach Team of I AM ALS. Kristin continues to work part time for the University of Illinois at Chicago School of Public Health, where she previously taught epidemiology methods and currently studies maternal and child health issues.

Julian (Jules) Rodriguez is a 38-year-old husband and father who was diagnosed with ALS in 2020. Jules receives full-time care from his wife and partner, Maria Aleandra. Along with their son, Skyler, the Rodriguez family lives by the mantra and motto, "Right Here, Right Now," as they weather the multitude of challenges (emotional, physical, mental, and spiritual) that ALS brings.

living with ALS (Horton et al., 2018). ALS clinical trials often struggle to identify participants that meet eligibility criteria and therefore some trials are insufficiently enrolled and incapable of providing meaningful data. There is no comprehensive national registry of ALS, precluding meaningful assessment of overall trends in the health of people with ALS. Progress in therapeutics has been inconsistent and halting, and there is little to offer genetic carriers who are watching the clock on their own symptoms, often while caring for close relatives dying of the disease. Frustrated by the lack of significant progress, many individuals and families experiencing one of the most devastating diseases known to humankind are calling for major change.

There are bright spots in the national picture. The committee heard many times about the value of care and supports for people with ALS within the U.S. Department of Veterans Affairs (VA) system. In the short term, everyone living with a devastating progressive disease such as ALS deserves, at a minimum, what the VA provides—care that frees an individual and their families from financial devastation because of the need to pay for ventilators, accessible vans, and home modifications; care that proactively delivers the interventions and equipment one needs before or just when needed; and care planning and services landscape navigation that includes partnering with caregivers and family members who will be at the side of the individual with ALS. The committee recommends actions that Congress, the Centers for Medicare & Medicaid Services (CMS), private insurers, ALS nonprofits, and patient-serving associations can take quickly to remove barriers for people with ALS to receive care and services that improve quality of life.

These steps, while crucial, are not sufficient to make ALS a livable disease. Success requires significant advances in basic science, clinical care, and population health. Looking to the longer term, the committee appreciated the progress made in cancer and cystic fibrosis, based on a strong platform of sustainable, integrated, and coordinated systems of care and research. People living with ALS, caregivers, and genetic carriers deserve such a system too. To this end, the committee recommends that research and clinical care be coordinated across ALS community, regional, and comprehensive centers. As a condition for enhanced funding every clinical center should facilitate access to a meaningful national patient registry and allow patients access to research studies, including clinical trials. The committee recommends actions Congress, NIH, CMS, ALS multidisciplinary care leaders, and community-based providers can take to build an inclusive and integrated care and research system, improve racial and ethnic equity in ALS care and research, align reimbursement to achieve the goals of the new system, and bolster VA clinical care, research, education, and informatics resources to further improve the comprehensiveness and reach of care for veterans.

The committee also makes recommendations for basic and translational research. The ACT for ALS research strategy holds enormous promise, and the committee believes realizing the full potential of the ACT for ALS initiatives underway is necessary to achieve the goal of making ALS a livable disease in 10 years. As this report describes, an integrated and adequately funded ALS care and research system will be the foundation for introducing the new therapies these ACT for ALS initiatives are working to accelerate.

The committee recognized that some of its recommendations are not unique to ALS and could apply to a broader range of diseases. For example, barriers that people living with ALS and their caregivers face in obtaining appropriate and affordable care are the same barriers experienced by many patients with other chronic and devastating diseases who are having difficulties getting excellent care and negotiating with insurance companies. These recommendations are needed for ALS and could serve as a model or proof of concept for other disease areas.

The committee believes that no single entity can have ultimate accountability for coordinating all the recommendations in this report. However, entities to whom specific recommendations are directed should see this as a challenge to act. These entities can be the impetus for transforming the landscape of ALS care on which others can build. It will be incumbent on the ALS advocacy community working with people living with ALS, caregivers, genetic carriers, and more to push forward the committee's recommendations and create the momentum for change. The committee hopes the ALS advocacy community will work collaboratively and build a set of expectations around the recommendations in this report and how they need to be addressed. This will ultimately involve the ALS advocacy community working with Congress, CMS, NIH, FDA, researchers, health systems, clinicians, industry (drug developer and technology companies), and the people who are impacted by ALS every day.

REFERENCES

Al-Chalabi, A., and O. Hardiman. 2013. The epidemiology of ALS: A conspiracy of genes, environment and time. *Nat Rev Neurol* 9(11):617–628.

Al-Chalabi, A., F. Fang, M. F. Hanby, P. N. Leigh, C. E. Shaw, W. Ye, and F. Rijsdijk. 2010. An estimate of amyotrophic lateral sclerosis heritability using twin data. *J Neurol Neurosurg Psychiatry* 81(12):1324–1326.

ALS Assocation. 2021. *thinkALS™ for Faster Diagnosis.* https://www.als.org/thinkals (accessed May 1, 2024).

Andrew, A. S., T. A. Caller, R. Tandan, E. J. Duell, P. L. Henegan, N. C. Field, W. G. Bradley, and E. W. Stommel. 2017. Environmental and occupational exposures and amyotrophic lateral sclerosis in New England. *Neurodegener Dis* 17(2–3):110–116.

Andrew, A. S., C. Y. Chen, T. A. Caller, R. Tandan, P. L. Henegan, B. P. Jackson, B. P. Hall, W. G. Bradley, and E. W. Stommel. 2018. Toenail mercury levels are associated with amyotrophic lateral sclerosis risk. *Muscle Nerve* 58(1):36–41.

Andrew, A., J. Zhou, J. Gui, A. Harrison, X. Shi, M. Li, B. Guetti, R. Nathan, M. Tischbein, E. P. Pioro, E. Stommel, and W. Bradley. 2021a. Pesticides applied to crops and amyotrophic lateral sclerosis risk in the U.S. *Neurotoxicology* 87:128–135.

Andrew, A. S., W. G. Bradley, D. Peipert, T. Butt, K. Amoako, E. P. Pioro, R. Tandan, J. Novak, A. Quick, K. D. Pugar, K. Sawlani, B. Katirji, T. A. Hayes, P. Cazzolli, J. Gui, P. Mehta, D. K. Horton, and E. W. Stommel. 2021b. Risk factors for amyotrophic lateral sclerosis: A regional United States case-control study. *Muscle Nerve* 63(1):52–59.

Arthur, K. C., A. Calvo, T. R. Price, J. T. Geiger, A. Chiò, and B. J. Traynor. 2016. Projected increase in amyotrophic lateral sclerosis from 2015 to 2040. *Nature Communications* 7(1):12408.

Benatar, M., J. Wuu, P. M. Andersen, V. Lombardi, and A. Malaspina. 2018. Neurofilament light: A candidate biomarker of presymptomatic amyotrophic lateral sclerosis and phenoconversion. *Ann Neurol* 84(1):130–139.

Benatar, M., J. Wuu, P. M. Andersen, R. C. Bucelli, J. A. Andrews, M. Otto, N. A. Farahany, E. A. Harrington, W. Chen, A. A. Mitchell, T. Ferguson, S. Chew, L. Gedney, S. Oakley, J. Heo, S. Chary, L. Fanning, D. Graham, P. Sun, Y. Liu, J. Wong, and S. Fradette. 2022a. Design of a randomized, placebo-controlled, phase 3 trial of tofersen initiated in clinically presymptomatic sod1 variant carriers: The atlas study. *Neurotherapeutics* 19(4):1248–1258.

Benatar, M., J. Wuu, C. McHutchison, R. B. Postuma, B. F. Boeve, R. Petersen, C. A. Ross, H. Rosen, J. J. Arias, S. Fradette, M. P. McDermott, J. Shefner, C. Stanislaw, S. Abrahams, S. Cosentino, P. M. Andersen, R. S. Finkel, V. Granit, A. L. Grignon, J. D. Rohrer, C. T. McMillan, M. Grossman, A. Al-Chalabi, and M. R. Turner. 2022b. Preventing amyotrophic lateral sclerosis: Insights from pre-symptomatic neurodegenerative diseases. *Brain* 145(1):27–44.

Benatar, M., S. A. Goutman, K. A. Staats, E. L. Feldman, M. Weisskopf, E. Talbott, K. D. Dave, N. M. Thakur, and A. Al-Chalabi. 2023. A roadmap to ALS prevention: Strategies and priorities. *J Neurol Neurosurg Psychiatry* 94(5):399–402.

Blank, R. H., J. B. Kurent, and D. Oliver. 2021. *Public policy in ALS/MND care: An international perspective*. New York: Palgrave Macmillan.

Boddy, S. L., I. Giovannelli, M. Sassani, J. Cooper-Knock, M. P. Snyder, E. Segal, E. Elinav, L. A. Barker, P. J. Shaw, and C. J. McDermott. 2021. The gut microbiome: A key player in the complexity of amyotrophic lateral sclerosis (ALS). *BMC Med* 19(1):13.

Brizzi, K. T., J. F. P. Bridges, J. Yersak, C. Balas, N. Thakur, M. Galvin, O. Hardiman, C. Heatwole, J. Ravits, Z. Simmons, L. Bruijn, J. Chan, R. Bedlack, and J. D. Berry. 2020. Understanding the needs of people with ALS: A national survey of patients and caregivers. *Amyotroph Lateral Scler Frontotemporal Degener* 21(5–6):355–363.

Chia, R., A. Chiò, and B. J. Traynor. 2018. Novel genes associated with amyotrophic lateral sclerosis: Diagnostic and clinical implications. *Lancet Neurology* 17(1):94–102.

Chiò, A., G. Logroscino, O. Hardiman, R. Swingler, D. Mitchell, E. Beghi, and B. G. Traynor. 2009. Prognostic factors in ALS: A critical review. *Amyotroph Lateral Scler* 10(5–6): 310–323.

Chiò, A., G. Mora, and G. Lauria. 2017. Pain in amyotrophic lateral sclerosis. *Lancet Neurol* 16(2):144–157.

Chiò, A., L. Mazzini, S. D'Alfonso, L. Corrado, A. Canosa, C. Moglia, U. Manera, E. Bersano, M. Brunetti, M. Barberis, J. H. Veldink, L. H. van den Berg, N. Pearce, W. Sproviero, R. McLaughlin, A. Vajda, O. Hardiman, J. Rooney, G. Mora, A. Calvo, and A. Al-Chalabi. 2018. The multistep hypothesis of ALS revisited: The role of genetic mutations. *Neurology* 91(7):e635–e642.

C-Path (Critical Path Institute). 2024. Rare neurodegenerative disease efforts under the ACT for ALS. https://www.youtube.com/watch?v=ugzCROY3-jA (accessed April 22, 2024).

C-Path. n.d. *Critical path for rare neurodegenerative diseases.* https://c-path.org/program/critical-path-for-rare-neurodegenerative-diseases (accessed April 22, 2024).

Cragg, J. J., N. J. Johnson, and M. G. Weisskopf. 2017. Military service and amyotrophic lateral sclerosis in a population-based cohort: Extended follow-up 1979–2011. *Epidemiology* 28(2):e15–e16.

Di Gioia, D., N. Bozzi Cionci, L. Baffoni, A. Amoruso, M. Pane, L. Mogna, F. Gaggìa, M. A. Lucenti, E. Bersano, R. Cantello, F. De Marchi, and L. Mazzini. 2020. A prospective longitudinal study on the microbiota composition in amyotrophic lateral sclerosis. *BMC Med* 18(1):153.

Dou, J., K. Bakulski, K. Guo, J. Hur, L. Zhao, S. Saez-Atienzar, A. Stark, R. Chia, A. García-Redondo, R. Rojas-Garcia, J. F. Vázquez Costa, R. Fernandez Santiago, S. Bandres-Ciga, P. Gómez-Garre, M. T. Periñán, P. Mir, J. Pérez-Tur, F. Cardona, M. Menendez-Gonzalez, J. Riancho, D. Borrego-Hernández, L. Galán-Dávila, J. Infante Ceberio, P. Pastor, C. Paradas, O. Dols-Icardo, B. J. Traynor, E. L. Feldman, and S. A. Goutman. 2023. Cumulative genetic score and c9orf72 repeat status independently contribute to amyotrophic lateral sclerosis risk in 2 case-control studies. *Neurol Genet* 9(4):e200079.

FDA (U.S. Food and Drug Administration). 2013. *Orphan Drug Act—relevant excerpts.* https://www.fda.gov/industry/designating-orphan-product-drugs-and-biological-products/orphan-drug-act-relevant-excerpts (accessed April 1, 2024).

FDA. 2024. *Accelerating access to critical therapies for ALS Act—ACT for ALS.* https://www.fda.gov/news-events/public-health-focus/accelerating-access-critical-therapies-als-act-act-als (accessed April 22, 2024).

Feldman, E. L., S. A. Goutman, S. Petri, L. Mazzini, M. G. Savelieff, P. J. Shaw, and G. Sobue. 2022. Amyotrophic lateral sclerosis. *Lancet* 400(10360):1363–1380.

Ferrari, R., D. Kapogiannis, E. D. Huey, and P. Momeni. 2011. FTD and ALS: A tale of two diseases. *Curr Alzheimer Res* 8(3):273–294.

Figueroa-Romero, C., K. A. Mikhail, C. Gennings, P. Curtin, G. A. Bello, T. M. Botero, S. A. Goutman, E. L. Feldman, M. Arora, and C. Austin. 2020. Early life metal dysregulation in amyotrophic lateral sclerosis. *Ann Clin Transl Neurol* 7(6):872–882.

Filippini, T., M. Fiore, M. Tesauro, C. Malagoli, M. Consonni, F. Violi, E. Arcolin, L. Iacuzio, G. Oliveri Conti, A. Cristaldi, P. Zuccarello, E. Zucchi, L. Mazzini, F. Pisano, I. Gagliardi, F. Patti, J. Mandrioli, M. Ferrante, and M. Vinceti. 2020a. Clinical and lifestyle factors and risk of amyotrophic lateral sclerosis: A population-based case-control study. *Int J Environ Res Public Health* 17(3).

Filippini, T., M. Tesauro, M. Fiore, C. Malagoli, M. Consonni, F. Violi, L. Iacuzio, E. Arcolin, G. Oliveri Conti, A. Cristaldi, P. Zuccarello, E. Zucchi, L. Mazzini, F. Pisano, I. Gagliardi, F. Patti, J. Mandrioli, M. Ferrante, and M. Vinceti. 2020b. Environmental and occupational risk factors of amyotrophic lateral sclerosis: A population-based case-control study. *Int J Environ Res Public Health* 17(8).

FNIH (Foundation for the National Institutes of Health). 2023. *Accelerating Medicines Partnership (AMP).* https://fnih.org/our-programs/accelerating-medicines-partnership-amp (accessed May 21, 2024).

FNIH. 2024. *AMP amyotrophic lateral sclerosis (ALS).* https://fnih.org/our-programs/accelerating-medicines-partnership-amp-amp-amyotrophic-lateral-sclerosis-als (accessed April 22, 2024).

Fontana, A., B. Marin, J. Luna, E. Beghi, G. Logroscino, F. Boumédiene, P. M. Preux, P. Couratier, and M. Copetti. 2021. Time-trend evolution and determinants of sex ratio in amyotrophic lateral sclerosis: A dose-response meta-analysis. *J Neurol* 268(8):2973–2984.

Goutman, S. A. 2017. Diagnosis and clinical management of amyotrophic lateral sclerosis and other motor neuron disorders. *Continuum (Minneapolis, Minn.)* 23(5, Peripheral Nerve and Motor Neuron Disorders):1332–1359.

Goutman, S. A., J. Boss, A. Patterson, B. Mukherjee, S. Batterman, and E. L. Feldman. 2019. High plasma concentrations of organic pollutants negatively impact survival in amyotrophic lateral sclerosis. *J Neurol Neurosurg Psychiatry* 90(8):907–912.

Goutman, S. A., J. Boss, C. Godwin, B. Mukherjee, E. L. Feldman, and S. A. Batterman. 2022a. Associations of self-reported occupational exposures and settings to ALS: A case-control study. *Int Arch Occup Environ Health* 95(7):1567–1586.

Goutman, S. A., J. Boss, C. Godwin, B. Mukherjee, E. L. Feldman, and S. A. Batterman. 2022b. Occupational history associates with ALS survival and onset segment. *Amyotroph Lateral Scler Frontotemporal Degener* 1–11.

Goutman, S. A., J. Boss, G. Iyer, H. Habra, M. G. Savelieff, A. Karnovsky, B. Mukherjee, and E. L. Feldman. 2022c. Body mass index associates with amyotrophic lateral sclerosis survival and metabolomic profiles. *Muscle Nerve* 67(3):208–216.

Goutman, S. A., O. Hardiman, A. Al-Chalabi, A. Chió, M. G. Savelieff, M. C. Kiernan, and E. L. Feldman. 2022d. Emerging insights into the complex genetics and pathophysiology of amyotrophic lateral sclerosis. *Lancet Neurol* 21(5):465–479.

Goutman, S. A., O. Hardiman, A. Al-Chalabi, A. Chió, M. G. Savelieff, M. C. Kiernan, and E. L. Feldman. 2022e. Recent advances in the diagnosis and prognosis of amyotrophic lateral sclerosis. *Lancet Neurol* 21(5):480–493.

Goutman, S. A., M. G. Savelieff, D. G. Jang, J. Hur, and E. L. Feldman. 2023. The amyotrophic lateral sclerosis exposome: Recent advances and future directions. *Nat Rev Neurol* 19(10):617–634.

Goutman, S. A., J. Boss, D. G. Jang, B. Mukherjee, R. J. Richardson, S. Batterman, and E. L. Feldman. 2024. Environmental risk scores of persistent organic pollutants associate with higher ALS risk and shorter survival in a new Michigan case/control cohort. *J Neurol Neurosurg Psychiatry* 95(3):241–248.

Gowland, A., S. Opie-Martin, K. M. Scott, A. R. Jones, P. R. Mehta, C. J. Batts, C. M. Ellis, P. N. Leigh, C. E. Shaw, J. Sreedharan, and A. Al-Chalabi. 2019. Predicting the future of ALS: The impact of demographic change and potential new treatments on the prevalence of ALS in the United Kingdom, 2020–2116. *Amyotroph Lateral Scler Frontotemporal Degener* 20(3–4):264–274.

Henry, K. A., J. Fagliano, H. M. Jordan, L. Rechtman, and W. E. Kaye. 2015. Geographic variation of amyotrophic lateral sclerosis incidence in New Jersey, 2009–2011. *Am J Epidemiol* 182(6):512–519.

Hertzberg, V. S., H. Singh, C. N. Fournier, A. Moustafa, M. Polak, C. A. Kuelbs, M. G. Torralba, M. G. Tansey, K. E. Nelson, and J. D. Glass. 2022. Gut microbiome differences between amyotrophic lateral sclerosis patients and spouse controls. *Amyotroph Lateral Scler Frontotemporal Degener* 23(1–2):91–99.

HHS (U.S. Department of Health and Human Services). 2023. *Amyotrophic lateral sclerosis (ALS) intermediate patient population expanded access (UO1 clinical trial required)*. https://grants.nih.gov/grants/guide/rfa-files/RFA-NS-24-029.html (accessed May 21, 2024).

Ho, D. T., R. Ruthazer, and J. A. Russell. 2011. Shoulder pain in amyotrophic lateral sclerosis. *J Clin Neuromuscul Dis* 13(1):53–55.

Horton, D. K., S. Graham, R. Punjani, G. Wilt, W. Kaye, K. Maginnis, L. Webb, J. Richman, R. Bedlack, E. Tessaro, and P. Mehta. 2018. A spatial analysis of amyotrophic lateral sclerosis (ALS) cases in the United States and their proximity to multidisciplinary ALS clinics, 2013. *Amyotroph Lateral Scler Frontotemporal Degener* 19(1–2):126–133.

Jaafar, N., E. Malek, H. Ismail, and J. Salameh. 2021. Nonmotor symptoms in amyotrophic lateral sclerosis and their correlation with disease progression. *J Clin Neuromuscul Dis* 23(1):1–6.

Jellinger, K. A. 2023. The spectrum of cognitive dysfunction in amyotrophic lateral sclerosis: An update. *Int J Mol Sci* 24(19).

Koeman, T., P. Slottje, L. J. Schouten, S. Peters, A. Huss, J. H. Veldink, H. Kromhout, P. A. van den Brandt, and R. Vermeulen. 2017. Occupational exposure and amyotrophic lateral sclerosis in a prospective cohort. *Occup Environ Med* 74(8):578–585.

Longinetti, E., and F. Fang. 2019. Epidemiology of amyotrophic lateral sclerosis: An update of recent literature. *Curr Opin Neurol* 32(5):771–776.

Luna, J., J. P. Leleu, P. M. Preux, P. Corcia, P. Couratier, B. Marin, and F. Boumediene. 2019. Residential exposure to ultra high frequency electromagnetic fields emitted by global system for mobile (GSM) antennas and amyotrophic lateral sclerosis incidence: A geo-epidemiological population-based study. *Environ Res* 176:108525.

Marin, B., F. Boumediene, G. Logroscino, P. Couratier, M. C. Babron, A. L. Leutenegger, M. Copetti, P. M. Preux, and E. Beghi. 2017. Variation in worldwide incidence of amyotrophic lateral sclerosis: A meta-analysis. *Int J Epidemiol* 46(1):57–74.

McCann, E. P., K. L. Williams, J. A. Fifita, I. S. Tarr, J. O'Connor, D. B. Rowe, G. A. Nicholson, and I. P. Blair. 2017. The genotype-phenotype landscape of familial amyotrophic lateral sclerosis in Australia. *Clin Genet* 92(3):259–266.

McKay, K. A., K. A. Smith, L. Smertinaite, F. Fang, C. Ingre, and F. Taube. 2021. Military service and related risk factors for amyotrophic lateral sclerosis. *Acta Neurol Scand* 143(1):39–50.

Mehta, P., J. Raymond, Y. Zhang, R. Punjani, M. Han, T. Larson, O. Muravov, R. H. Lyles, and D. K. Horton. 2023. Prevalence of amyotrophic lateral sclerosis in the United States, 2018. *Amyotroph Lateral Scler Frontotemporal Degener* 24(7–8):702–708.

Miller, R. G., C. E. Jackson, E. J. Kasarskis, J. D. England, D. Forshew, M. Johnston, K. Kalra, J. S. Katz, H. Mitsumoto, J. Rosenfeld, C. Shoesmith, M. J. Strong, and S. C. Woolley. 2009. Practice parameter update: The care of the patient with amyotrophic lateral sclerosis: Multidisciplinary care, symptom management, and cognitive/behavioral impairment (an evidence-based review). Report of the Quality Standards Subcommittee of the American Academy of Neurology. *Neurology* 73(15):1227–1233.

Myung, W., H. Lee, and H. Kim. 2019. Short-term air pollution exposure and emergency department visits for amyotrophic lateral sclerosis: A time-stratified case-crossover analysis. *Environ Int* 123:467–475.

NASEM (National Academies of Sciences, Engineering, and Medicine). 2023. *Amyotrophic lateral sclerosis: Accelerating treatments and improving quality of life: Proceedings of a workshop—in brief.* Washington, DC: The National Academies Press.

Newell, M. E., S. Adhikari, and R. U. Halden. 2022. Systematic and state-of the science review of the role of environmental factors in amyotrophic lateral sclerosis (ALS) or Lou Gehrig's disease. *Sci Total Environ* 817:152504.

Nicholson, K., A. Murphy, E. McDonnell, J. Shapiro, E. Simpson, J. Glass, H. Mitsumoto, D. Forshew, R. Miller, and N. Atassi. 2018. Improving symptom management for people with amyotrophic lateral sclerosis. *Muscle Nerve* 57(1):20–24.

Nicholson, K., K. Bjornevik, G. Abu-Ali, J. Chan, M. Cortese, B. Dedi, M. Jeon, R. Xavier, C. Huttenhower, A. Ascherio, and J. D. Berry. 2021. The human gut microbiota in people with amyotrophic lateral sclerosis. *Amyotroph Lateral Scler Frontotemporal Degener* 22(3–4):186–194.

NIH (National Institutes of Health). 2023. *Priorities of the NIH amyotrophic lateral sclerosis (ALS) strategic planning working group.* https://www.ninds.nih.gov/sites/default/files/documents/ALS%20Strategic%20Plan_01_19_23_508C_2.pdf (accessed April 23, 2024).

NIH. 2024. *Estimates of funding for various research, condition, and disease categories (RCDC).* https://report.nih.gov/funding/categorical-spending (accessed May 21, 2024).

NINDS (National Institute of Neurological Disorders and Stroke). 2023a. *NIH implementation of ACT for ALS.* https://www.ninds.nih.gov/news-events/news/highlights-announcements/nih-implementation-act-als (accessed April 22, 2024).

NINDS. 2023b. *ACT for ALS & ALS strategic priorities community update*. https://www. ninds.nih.gov/news-events/events/act-als-als-strategic-priorities-community-update (accessed April 22, 2024).

Nunez, Y., A. K. Boehme, J. Goldsmith, M. Li, A. van Donkelaar, M. G. Weisskopf, D. B. Re, R. V. Martin, and M. A. Kioumourtzoglou. 2022. PM(2.5) composition and disease aggravation in amyotrophic lateral sclerosis: An analysis of long-term exposure to components of fine particulate matter in New York State. *Environ Epidemiol* 6(2):e204.

Parks, R. M., Y. Nunez, A. A. Balalian, E. A. Gibson, J. Hansen, O. Raaschou-Nielsen, M. Ketzel, J. Khan, J. Brandt, R. Vermeulen, S. Peters, J. Goldsmith, D. B. Re, M. G. Weisskopf, and M. A. Kioumourtzoglou. 2022. Long-term traffic-related air pollutant exposure and amyotrophic lateral sclerosis diagnosis in Denmark: A Bayesian hierarchical analysis. *Epidemiology* 33(6):757–766.

Peters, T. L., F. Kamel, C. Lundholm, M. Feychting, C. E. Weibull, D. P. Sandler, P. Wiebert, P. Sparen, W. Ye, and F. Fang. 2017. Occupational exposures and the risk of amyotrophic lateral sclerosis. *Occup Environ Med* 74(2):87–92.

Peters, S., A. E. Visser, F. D'Ovidio, E. Beghi, A. Chiò, G. Logroscino, O. Hardiman, H. Kromhout, A. Huss, J. Veldink, R. Vermeulen, L. H. van den Berg, and M. C. Euro. 2019. Associations of electric shock and extremely low-frequency magnetic field exposure with the risk of amyotrophic lateral sclerosis. *Am J Epidemiol* 188(4):796–805.

Peters, S., A. E. Visser, F. D'Ovidio, J. Vlaanderen, L. Portengen, E. Beghi, A. Chiò, G. Logroscino, O. Hardiman, E. Pupillo, J. H. Veldink, R. Vermeulen, and L. H. van den Berg. 2020. Effect modification of the association between total cigarette smoking and ALS risk by intensity, duration and time-since-quitting: Euro-motor. *J Neurol Neurosurg Psychiatry* 91(1):33–39.

Peters, S., K. Broberg, V. Gallo, M. Levi, M. Kippler, P. Vineis, J. Veldink, L. van den Berg, L. Middleton, R. C. Travis, M. M. Bergmann, D. Palli, S. Grioni, R. Tumino, A. Elbaz, T. Vlaar, F. Mancini, T. Kuhn, V. Katzke, A. Agudo, F. Goni, J. H. Gomez, M. Rodriguez-Barranco, S. Merino, A. Barricarte, A. Trichopoulou, M. Jenab, E. Weiderpass, and R. Vermeulen. 2021. Blood metal levels and amyotrophic lateral sclerosis risk: A prospective cohort. *Ann Neurol* 89(1):125–133.

Pupillo, E., M. Poloni, E. Bianchi, G. Giussani, G. Logroscino, S. Zoccolella, A. Chiò, A. Calvo, M. Corbo, C. Lunetta, B. Marin, D. Mitchell, O. Hardiman, J. Rooney, Z. Stevic, M. Bandettini di Poggio, M. Filosto, M. S. Cotelli, M. Perini, N. Riva, L. Tremolizzo, E. Vitelli, D. Damiani, E. Beghi, and EURALS Consortium. 2018. Trauma and amyotrophic lateral sclerosis: A European population-based case-control study from the EURALS Consortium. *Amyotroph Lateral Scler Frontotemporal Degener* 19(1–2):118–125.

Richards, D., J. A. Morren, and E. P. Pioro. 2021. Time to diagnosis and factors affecting diagnostic delay in amyotrophic lateral sclerosis. In *Amyotrophic lateral sclerosis*, edited by T. Araki. Brisbane, Australia: Exon Publications.

Sagiraju, H. K. R., S. Živković, A. C. VanCott, H. Patwa, D. Gimeno Ruiz de Porras, M. E. Amuan, and M. J. V. Pugh. 2020. Amyotrophic lateral sclerosis among veterans deployed in support of post-9/11 U.S. conflicts. *Mil Med* 185(3–4):e501–e509.

Seelen, M., R. A. Toro Campos, J. H. Veldink, A. E. Visser, G. Hoek, B. Brunekreef, A. J. van der Kooi, M. de Visser, J. Raaphorst, L. H. van den Berg, and R. C. H. Vermeulen. 2017. Long-term air pollution exposure and amyotrophic lateral sclerosis in the Netherlands: A population-based case-control study. *Environ Health Perspect* 125(9):097023.

Simmons, Z. 2015. Patient-perceived outcomes and quality of life in ALS. *Neurotherapeutics* 12(2):394–402.

Souza, P. V. S., P. L. Serrano, I. B. Farias, R. I. L. Machado, B. M. L. Badia, H. B. Oliveira, A. S. Barbosa, C. A. Pereira, V. F. Moreira, M. A. T. Chieia, A. R. Barbosa, V. L. Braga, W. Pinto, and A. S. B. Oliveira. 2024. Clinical and genetic aspects of juvenile amyotrophic lateral sclerosis: A promising era emerges. *Genes* 15(3).

Su, F. C., S. A. Goutman, S. Chernyak, B. Mukherjee, B. C. Callaghan, S. Batterman, and E. L. Feldman. 2016. Association of environmental toxins with amyotrophic lateral sclerosis. *JAMA Neurol* 73(7):803–811.

Thakore, N. J., B. R. Lapin, H. Mitsumoto, and C. Pooled Resource Open-Access Als Clinical Trials. 2022. Early initiation of riluzole may improve absolute survival in amyotrophic lateral sclerosis. *Muscle Nerve* 66(6):702–708.

Turner, M. R., J. Barnwell, A. Al-Chalabi, and A. Eisen. 2012. Young-onset amyotrophic lateral sclerosis: Historical and other observations. *Brain* 135(Pt 9):2883–2891.

van Rheenen, W., A. Shatunov, A. M. Dekker, R. L. McLaughlin, F. P. Diekstra, S. L. Pulit, R. A. van der Spek, et al. 2016. Genome-wide association analyses identify new risk variants and the genetic architecture of amyotrophic lateral sclerosis. *Nat Genet* 48(9):1043–1048.

Vasta, R., F. D'Ovidio, A. Canosa, U. Manera, M. C. Torrieri, M. Grassano, F. De Marchi, L. Mazzini, C. Moglia, A. Calvo, and A. Chiò. 2020. Plateaus in amyotrophic lateral sclerosis progression: Results from a population-based cohort. *Eur J Neurol* 27(8):1397–1404.

Wang, M. D., J. Little, J. Gomes, N. R. Cashman, and D. Krewski. 2017. Identification of risk factors associated with onset and progression of amyotrophic lateral sclerosis using systematic review and meta-analysis. *Neurotoxicology* 61:101–130.

Westeneng, H. J., T. P. A. Debray, A. E. Visser, R. P. A. van Eijk, J. P. K. Rooney, A. Calvo, S. Martin, C. J. McDermott, A. G. Thompson, S. Pinto, X. Kobeleva, A. Rosenbohm, B. Stubendorff, H. Sommer, B. M. Middelkoop, A. M. Dekker, J. van Vugt, W. van Rheenen, A. Vajda, M. Heverin, M. Kazoka, H. Hollinger, M. Gromicho, S. Korner, T. M. Ringer, A. Rodiger, A. Gunkel, C. E. Shaw, A. L. Bredenoord, M. A. van Es, P. Corcia, P. Couratier, M. Weber, J. Grosskreutz, A. C. Ludolph, S. Petri, M. de Carvalho, P. Van Damme, K. Talbot, M. R. Turner, P. J. Shaw, A. Al-Chalabi, A. Chio, O. Hardiman, K. G. M. Moons, J. H. Veldink, and L. H. van den Berg. 2018. Prognosis for patients with amyotrophic lateral sclerosis: Development and validation of a personalised prediction model. *Lancet Neurol* 17(5):423–433.

Westeneng, H. J., K. van Veenhuijzen, R. A. van der Spek, S. Peters, A. E. Visser, W. van Rheenen, J. H. Veldink, and L. H. van den Berg. 2021. Associations between lifestyle and amyotrophic lateral sclerosis stratified by C9orf72 genotype: A longitudinal, population-based, case-control study. *Lancet Neurol* 20(5):373–384.

Wijesekera, L. C., and P. Nigel Leigh. 2009. Amyotrophic lateral sclerosis. *Orphanet: J Rare Dis* 4(1):3.

Wolf, J., A. Safer, J. C. Wöhrle, F. Palm, W. A. Nix, M. Maschke, and A. J. Grau. 2014. Factors predicting one-year mortality in amyotrophic lateral sclerosis patients—data from a population-based registry. *BMC Neurology* 14(1):197.

Xu, L., T. Liu, L. Liu, X. Yao, L. Chen, D. Fan, S. Zhan, and S. Wang. 2020. Global variation in prevalence and incidence of amyotrophic lateral sclerosis: A systematic review and meta-analysis. *J Neurol* 267(4):944–953.

2

Living with ALS Today

ABSTRACT

One element in this study's statement of task is to articulate what would be needed to make amyotrophic lateral sclerosis (ALS) a livable disease in a decade. As a tool to help respond to that task, the committee uses this chapter as an attempt to describe what it means to live with ALS today. There is no one definition of livability in the context of ALS, given that every person living with ALS, every person with a genetic risk of developing ALS, and every family member of someone with ALS has their own unique experience living with the disease. However, it is clear from speaking with people living with ALS or with a genetic risk of developing ALS and their family members that there are addressable challenges and barriers that make living with ALS far more difficult that it needs to be. As discussed in this chapter, a big step toward making ALS a livable disease would include minimizing (1) the day-to-day challenges confronting people living with ALS, (2) the difficulty obtaining the necessary care and services, (3) the emotional and mental health toll of having a progressively disabling and invariably fatal disease, and (4) the economic burden that can devastate a family's finances.

Guaranteeing equitable access to high-quality, multidisciplinary care for all individuals, regardless of socioeconomic status or geographical location, is of paramount importance. This would include providing affordable and equitable access to physical, occupational, speech, respiratory, and behavioral therapies; durable medical equipment, such as electric wheelchairs and noninvasive ventilators; and palliative care, all without having to prove present or future necessity, given the diagnosis of ALS. Eliminating the substantial delay many if not most people with ALS experience in getting a clear diagnosis is critically important, both to start multidisciplinary care as soon as possible and to alleviate the substantial emotional burden that comes with waiting and uncertainty. This requires better educating primary care physicians and general neurologists about ALS and its many presentations. These are all achievable in the near term and would help realize the goal of making ALS a livable disease within a decade.

MAKING ALS LIVABLE IN 10 YEARS

To address the charge of providing recommendations to make ALS livable in 10 years, the committee worked to define making the disease "livable." In the committee's own discussions, and in discussions with people living with ALS, the committee realized that making it livable has two important, primary dimensions: (1) increasing the effectiveness of treatment, with the goal of managing symptoms, increasing longevity and ultimately finding a cure; and (2) increasing the quality of life, as measured by the level of satisfaction and enjoyment experienced by people with ALS. This means that ALS is livable when an individual diagnosed with ALS or at genetic risk of developing ALS can survive, thrive, and live a long, meaningful life while meeting the medical, psychosocial, and economic challenges of the disease. Combining these elements into a single definition has several important implications.

First, making ALS livable means accelerating efforts to find effective treatments for ALS. This is likely to require discoveries in the pathogenesis of the disease, the development of effective biomarkers, a more responsive and effective clinical trials network, and other steps, as outlined in Chapters 5 and 6.

Second, making ALS livable means helping all people with ALS and their families receive the current standard of care. Today, that standard is multidisciplinary care in clinics that can provide prompt diagnosis and essential care. To this end, Chapters 3 and 4 outline a series of recommendations for developing a more effective clinic structure to reach all Americans with ALS and at-risk ALS genetic carriers as well as closing policy gaps that make it hard for people with ALS to receive what they need.

Third, making ALS livable means addressing the social, economic, and mental health stresses associated with this devastating disease. Chapter 3 discusses policies to support family caregivers, prevent unnecessary expenses, and enhance mental health services.

Fourth, and finally, to make this dual definition of making ALS livable work, it is necessary to measure progress in both longevity and quality of life at the population level. It is not possible to answer whether ALS is becoming more livable by hearing about one person, or even 1,000. ALS is only becoming more livable if people with ALS in the aggregate are living longer and if their lives are more satisfying and fulfilling. It is telling that even baseline data for the current state of the ALS population do not exist. Assessment of these fundamental questions requires population level data systems, such as a comprehensive registry, which is covered in Chapter 5. Once developed, it will be possible to assess where the population of persons with ALS now stand and to set specific goals.

Operationalizing Livability

There are many ways to operationalize what it means to make ALS a livable disease. The most obvious definition of what it means to make ALS a livable disease is to develop a cure or effective therapies capable of transforming ALS from a fatal disease into a chronic one with easily managed symptoms that have little effect on the quality of life for people living with ALS, their family members, and other caregivers. In the time until a cure is developed, measurable, actionable goals are needed to ensure progress is made. One possibility is to focus on monitoring 5- and 10-year survival rates for individuals with ALS and compare to what is currently known about long-term cumulative survival in ALS to understand progress made and improvements still needed.

Regardless of metric, people with ALS deserve to be able to live long and fulfilling lives, unhampered by the progression of this disease. The committee believes increases in survival are possible if, while a cure and meaningful treatments for ALS are being pursued, there is also a renewed focus on improving clinical outcomes and quality of life, beginning with the interventions and care services available today. For example, it is unknown how many individuals with ALS are receiving the critical, first line medical treatment (riluzole) early on in their diagnosis. Estimates indicate a range of 38 percent (MDA, 2018) to 72 percent of persons with ALS in the United States receive riluzole (Takei et al., 2017). To do better for people living with ALS, a more complete, accurate picture of how the population is doing and the treatments they are receiving is needed. There are also many care services and interventions that help people with ALS live better and longer. For example, reducing diagnostic delay, the early initiation of noninvasive ventilation, and the use of multidisciplinary care have significant effects on both survival and quality of life (de Almeida et al., 2021; Gwathmey et al., 2023; Witzel et al., 2022). Support services such as nutritional care, palliative care, and mental health care have also demonstrated encouraging effects as well (Ludolph et al., 2023; Rosa Silva et al., 2020; Wu et al., 2022). More universal application of interventions known to improve prognosis for people with ALS, earlier initiation of these interventions, and continued research into how to make them most effective would create immediate impact for people living with ALS and their caregivers.

Pursuit of any metric focused on clinical outcomes needs to be pursued in parallel with robust efforts to improve quality of life to make ALS a livable disease in the next 10 years. There are many measurements of quality of life that can and are used in ALS today. The committee envisions that quality-of-life measures would capture the ability of an individual with ALS to do what is meaningful for them. ALS is livable when the individual is confident they can pursue and achieve what for them in life has meaning and to avoid financial devastation in doing so. Sources for meaning can include work, personal relationships, and improving the lives of others with ALS. These are more likely to be achieved when there is expedited access to essential ALS medical and support services; centralized resources to receive support for needs not otherwise accessible or covered by insurance; proper training and compensation of caregivers; access to therapies and technologies that prolong life, improving quality and function; maintenance of financial stability; and preventing ALS in at-risk persons. For people at genetic risk of developing ALS, having measures that prevent the onset of life-altering symptoms would make ALS a livable disease.

The committee held public discussions with people living with ALS, people at genetic risk of developing ALS, and the individuals who care for and treat people with ALS (see Boxes 2-1 and 2-2). No two people experience ALS the same way. As their disease develops, their priorities and aspects of life they focus on may change. Regardless of their individual priorities and focus, making aspects of day-to-day life more accessible to people living with ALS would greatly improve their quality of life. Achieving this requires making care, equipment, and other resources more widely accessible for everyone living with ALS, regardless of who they are and where they live. Individuals with ALS who know that drugs, devices, and supportive services can likely address future inevitable symptoms will live better today. For example, having that knowledge can lessen the anxiety and depression that often accompanies an uncertain future with ALS and can allow a person living with ALS to anticipate that they can continue to find meaning and participate in life.

Challenges to Improving Livability

A diagnosis of ALS is life changing for individuals and their families, and having timely access to high-quality, affordable treatment is imperative to easing the transitions that accompany an ALS diagnosis. The symptoms

BOX 2-1
Perspectives on Living with ALS

"Living well with ALS sounds counterintuitive . . . but those of us who have it have to try to do the best we can with it . . . trying to live well is constantly trying to be comfortable and have the resources we need to accommodate the myriad of needs that I have. . . . Some would say just living is a good thing. Well, at least you're alive. Yes, that's nice, but I think it's more about to be able to be useful and do things that help others. That's part of how I live well—by writing on a regular basis about ALS."
—Jim Clingman, person living with ALS[a]

"For me, living well is living the fight against the disease. I go to ball games, I go to bars, I go out for dinner or brunches with friends like I used to. . . . It's probably going to kill me, but if I'm successful working with everyone else with this disease who's engaged in the fight, it may kill me first but I'm going to kill it in the end. Me and everybody else. That's my mission, and that's my living with it. My living with it is my killing it."
—Paul Seifert, person living with ALS[a]

"It is so scary, but you can get through it. Find a good clinic, find a community, and ask for help. Many tools help me live my best life. My comfortable wheelchair, my Tobii Dynavox, which allows me to control everything around me, the bipap I wear at night to get a restful night's sleep and wake up refreshed and ready to attack the day. But you can still find meaning living with ALS."
—Desiree Galvez Kessler, person living with ALS[a]

Asia was diagnosed with ALS in 2016, yet she never let anything steal her shine or her zest for travel. Since diagnosis, Asia has traveled throughout the United States and been to Greece, Thailand, Mexico, the Bahamas, and the Dominican Republic. Asia created #AsiaDay in July 2020 where she does everything her heart desires, including a 90-minute massage, shopping, new restaurants, live events, or searching for the perfect mojito.
—Asia Jami, person living with ALS[a]

---

[a] Presented by Jim Clingman, Paul Seifert, Desiree Galvez Kessler, Asia Jami, and Kristin Rankin at "Amyotrophic Lateral Sclerosis: Accelerating Treatments and Improving Quality of Life – public workshop" on August 23, 2023; Asia Jami's comment is a brief biography that was read out by study staff during the workshop.

continued

BOX 2-1 Continued

"Some may ask how one can look at an ALS diagnosis and see anything that could be called a 'positive change.' In my case, continually looking for positives is a large part of what has kept me going for the last 6 years. . . . I have been active in ALS research . . . through my involvement in clinical trials, expanded access programs, and observational research studies, I have met some truly amazing and dedicated researchers. For the last 2 years, I have looked forward to spending a half-day at the hospital every 2 weeks getting an infusion of an experimental medication simply for the opportunity to spend time learning from people who are incredibly caring and empathetic."
—*Bruce D. Rosenblum, person with lived ALS experience*[b]

"Participating in a trial made me feel like I regained some control over my situation, like I was doing something to fight back against the disease, and it gave me hope, even though I didn't know if I was in the placebo or treatment group. It also feels good to contribute to moving the science along, which I've heard from other people living with ALS, too."
—*Kristin Rankin, person living with ALS*[c]

---

[b]Presented by Bruce Rosenblum at "Amyotrophic Lateral Sclerosis: Accelerating Treatments and Improving Quality of Life – public workshop" on August 10, 2023.
[c]Personal communication received by the committee on February 8, 2024.

---

of ALS often impede basic motor function and day-to-day activities, while less frequently, symptoms arise such as emotional difficulties and unusual behaviors associated with co-occurring frontotemporal dementia. People living with ALS must continually adapt their living environment to meet changing needs as the disease progresses.

> I immediately realized that we would have to move because there was no way our home could reasonably be made accessible, and my wife and I would have to sell the software business we had spent 25 years building.
> —*Bruce D. Rosenblum, person with lived ALS experience,*
> *presented during August 2023 public workshop*

Durable medical equipment (DME), home modification, and assistive technology can help with everyday activities and enable individuals with ALS and their families to minimize disruptions and maximize quality

---

BOX 2-2
Caregiver Views on Quality of Life

"Quality of life for my family meant maintaining some normalcy within the household and sticking to a routine as much as possible. He had a tracheostomy and ventilator, catheter, feeding tube. We would do whatever we had to, and he was ready to do whatever we had to so we could keep a normal family unit as much as possible."
—Siobhan Pandya, caregiver for a person living with ALS

"Our quality of life looked very different because Niesha was only 22 years old. To her, her quality of life was trying to accept what had happened and what was happening to her as a 22-year-old young adult, live with the fact that her body was changing, everything was changing and she didn't have any control over it, and make decisions for herself based on having a better quality of life."
—Vanessa Jackson, Mother/caregiver of person living/
passed away from ALS

SOURCE: Presented by Siobhan Pandya and Vanessa Jackson at "Amyotrophic Lateral Sclerosis: Accelerating Treatments and Improving Quality of Life – public workshop" on August 23, 2023.

---

of life. Home care, discussed in Chapter 3, becomes important as symptoms become more disabling, as is respite and mental health care for family members to help them deal with the emotional and physical stress of caring for an individual with ALS. However, unless a person with ALS is a veteran and receives care from the U.S. Department of Veterans Affairs (VA) (see Chapter 4), dealing with insurance challenges such as preauthorization requirements can make accessing DME, home modification, assistive technology, and home care a significant burden for individuals with ALS and their families (see Chapter 3 for more on insurance challenges).

ALS is a complex disease demanding a multidisciplinary approach to care involving a wide range of health care professionals and ancillary services. Box 2-3 lists some of the challenges and opportunities identified by the individuals with ALS and their families and caregivers that the committee consulted. The committee considered each issue and the opportunities to address them in its deliberations on how to make ALS a livable disease in the next decade. The recommendations the committee offers in

---

BOX 2-3
Action List for the ALS Community

The following is a list of some of the challenges and opportunities identified by the individuals with ALS, as well as their families and caregivers, who provided feedback to the committee:

For people living with ALS:

- a cure for ALS; currently there are only three treatments with limited efficacy
- equitable access to high-quality, multidisciplinary care for all individuals, regardless of socioeconomic status or geographical location
- implementing the U.S. Department of Veterans Affairs standard of care for all people living with ALS
- affordable access to physical therapy, occupational therapy, and speech therapy
- affordable access to respiratory therapy, including noninvasive ventilation
- affordable access to mental health services
- universal access to durable medical equipment, such as noninvasive ventilators and eye-tracking devices
- insurance coverage of electric wheelchairs; one chair can cost $25,000 out of pocket
- federal protections for aid-in-dying laws
- palliative care; hospice is not enough

---

subsequent chapters of this report seek to address many of these issues and catalyze large-scale system changes that would better serve individuals living with ALS, their families, and people at genetic risk of developing ALS for many decades into the future.

Diagnostic Delays

While advances have occurred over the past 20 years in understanding the genetic and environmental risk factors for ALS, delayed diagnosis remains a challenge (Falcão de Campos et al., 2021; Kraemer et al., 2010; Williams et al., 2013). Multiple studies have found the average delay from the first signs that something is wrong to confirmed diagnosis is 10 to 16 months. This is a significant length of time, considering the mean survival time with ALS is 2 to 5 years (see Table 2-1 and Figure 2-1) (Falcão de Campos et al., 2022; Galvin et al., 2015; Matharan et al., 2020a; Richards et al., 2021). Earlier diagnosis would

- reliable remote cognitive and physical testing
- education of primary care and primary neurologists about symptoms and early diagnosis
- a program to lessen the feeling of isolation

For caregivers:

- a strong program to lessen the feeling of isolation
- access to mental health services
- a way for working caregivers to avoid financial ruin when caring for a loved one
- paid respite care

For the genetic ALS community:

- enrollment in clinical trials
- protections against discrimination by employers and insurers

For the ALS community at large:

- increased research funding
- collection and sharing of biospecimens
- collaboration between hospitals, pharmaceutical companies, and nonprofit organizations
- a national registry including all people living with ALS and people at genetic risk of developing ALS

TABLE 2-1 Diagnostic Delay After Symptom Onset

	A. First Symptom to GP Visit	B. First Symptom to First Neuro	C. First Symptom to Diagnosis	D. First Symptom to MDC
Months	• ----5.5 months---->			
	• ----------------11.2 months---------------->			
	• --------------------------------16.0 months-------------------------------->			
	• --19.1 months-->			
Mean	5.5	11.2	16.0	19.1
Median	3.0	8.0	13.0	14.6
SD	6.8	8.4	9.5	11.6
Range	0–25	0–35	4–48	8–54
N	31	33	35	35

NOTE: GP = general practitioner; MDC = multidisciplinary care; N = sample size; SD = standard deviation.
SOURCE: Galvin et al., 2015. CC BY 4.0.

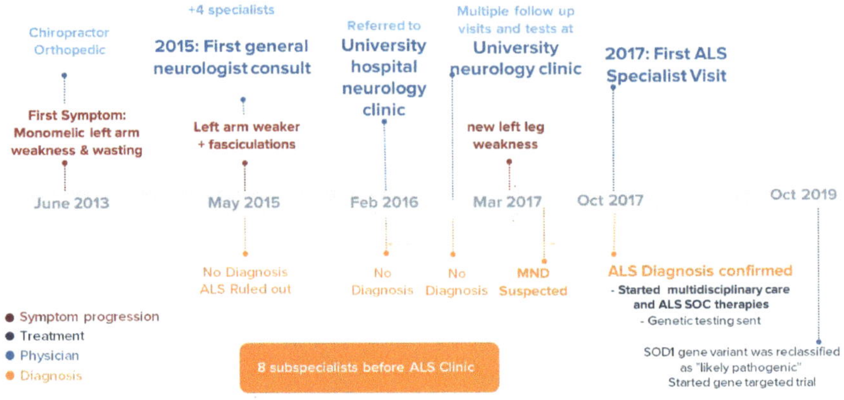

FIGURE 2-1 One individual's lived experience with diagnostic delay.
NOTE: MND = motor neuron disease; SOC = standard of care.
SOURCE: Babu et al., 2022, used with permission from Medscape, LLC © 2022.

enable an individual to start multidisciplinary care sooner,[1] which studies have shown can extend survival and improve quality of life (Hogden et al., 2017; Miller et al., 2009b; Ng et al., 2009). As new and potentially more effective ALS treatments are approved, earlier diagnosis becomes even more important. Timely diagnosis also allows people living with ALS and families time to prepare for the emotional trauma that accompanies an ALS diagnosis before the most debilitating symptoms develop (Paganoni et al., 2014).

However, research has suggested that individuals have an average of three consultations before receiving an ALS diagnosis, and nearly a quarter of ALS cases are first suspected by a physician other than a general neurologist or ALS specialist (Paganoni et al., 2014). Individuals who are Black, or who have a low income, and those who suffer cognitive impairment experience longer delays to diagnosis (Carter, 2022).

---

[1] The committee notes that interdisciplinary, rather than multidisciplinary, is the more accurate term because interdisciplinary denotes that the various disciplines are coordinated toward a common and coherent approach, while multidisciplinary refers to the addition of the competencies of multiple professionals who stay within the boundaries of their fields (Choi and Pak, 2006). The Veterans Health Administration refers to the ALS interdisciplinary team in its directive on providing ALS care to veterans. The committee has chosen to use multidisciplinary in the report because it is the more widely used term.

BOX 2-4
Diagnostic Delay in ALS

"My experience began in 2020 with a little problem with my right hand, and it progressed from there. My diagnosis didn't come until January of 2023, and it was kind of a shock, because I had a neurologist telling me that it was not ALS. So, when I got the genetic test result back, they told me I had it and that it was a particularly specific type of ALS. A mutation of the C9orf72 gene. It was a bit of a shock for two reasons. One, I had been getting told that it was something else. Ulnar neuropathy, spinal muscular atrophy, or they just didn't know. The other whammy was that because it is a dominant familial gene, I had to tell my three kids that I had a 50/50 chance of having passed it along to them, and that if they had it they would have a 50/50 chance of passing it on to their kids, my grandkids. It makes a difference to get treatment early, a big difference. Even though the medications out there are not terribly effective, the earlier you take them the more effective they are. I am somewhat hobbled by the fact that I'm late to the game on that."

—Paul Seifert, person living with ALS

"Jim was diagnosed with ALS the end of August 2013; however, he had symptoms 4 years prior, and he was misdiagnosed, actually. He had gone through long, extensive therapy because he was an avid cyclist, so thinking that it was a pinched nerve his surgeon did a laminectomy on him saying that is what his issue was. He was showing weakness in his lower left leg and riding with one leg practically. And he was bowling also in several leagues and falling all the time but not really understanding what was going on. It took 4 years for them to actually diagnose him."

—Sylvia Clingman, caregiver for a person living with ALS

SOURCE: Presented by Paul Seifert and Sylvia Clingman at "Amyotrophic Lateral Sclerosis: Accelerating Treatments and Improving Quality of Life - #2" on August 23, 2023.

Physician Factors in Diagnostic Delay

Diagnosing ALS may be challenging because of the rarity with which it is encountered in a nonneurology practice. A typical primary care physician may encounter individuals with ALS a handful of times in their career (Gwathmey et al., 2023). Awareness of the classic ALS presentation of difficulty swallowing and leg weakness may be inadequate, especially as the literature on ALS's heterogeneous presentation continues to develop.

If recognized, less common, nonmotor symptoms of ALS, such as executive dysfunction, cognitive decline, and neuropsychiatric symptoms, can improve the physician's diagnostic decision making.

A challenge for primary care clinicians is discerning when a patient with what appears to be an unusual presentation of a common disease, such as a pinched nerve root in the spinal cord, stroke, chronic obstructive pulmonary disease, or carpal tunnel syndrome, actually has ALS. The clinician's diagnostic skills may be tested further when a patient's newly emerging ALS is superimposed on an underlying chronic condition such as spinal stenosis.

> Only 2 years after I was diagnosed did I come to understand how fortunate I was with the diagnostic process. I was diagnosed in exactly 2 months; the average time to diagnose an ALS patient is 11 months. My initial [primary care physician] quickly focused on a neurologic issue based on the description in my email. When the lumbar MRI was negative, he immediately arranged for an EMG. The speed with which he ordered the EMG saved months of diagnostic time. He was never alarmist about the process and did not offer speculative diagnoses. Although it was difficult to first hear the term *ALS* when being diagnosed, I am grateful I didn't have to suffer with the knowledge that it was suspected throughout the 2-month diagnostic process.
>
> With incredible good fortune, both neurologists I saw were ALS specialists at ALS multidisciplinary centers. The first neurologist patiently gave us the time we needed that day, and he did not limit us to a 15-minute appointment when we clearly needed more. The appointment at the second hospital lasted 4 hours; we met with the neurologist, a physical therapist, and a research access nurse who talked with us about opportunities to participate in clinical trials.
>
> Having these two appointments 1 week apart was a blessing. By the end of the first appointment, we were too drained to absorb any more information. By the next week, we had the mental and emotional space to speak with the additional members of the [multidisciplinary care] team and start to develop an action and care plan.
>
> *—Bruce D. Rosenblum, person with lived ALS experience,*
> *presented during August 2023 public workshop*

The ALS Association's (ALSA's) thinkALS tool (see Figure 2-2), may help clinicians arrive at a timelier diagnosis (Gwathmey et al., 2023; Yersak et al., 2021). However, broader awareness of the tool's existence is needed. A challenge will be educating both nonneurology primary care providers and other specialists often consulted during the diagnostic odyssey, including orthopedists, otolaryngologists, rheumatologists, and pulmonary physicians.

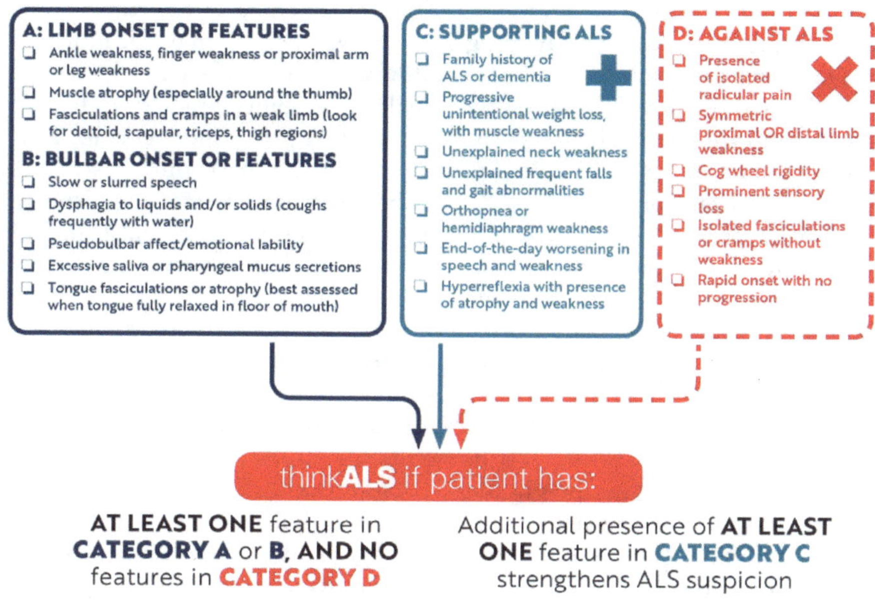

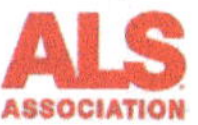

FIGURE 2-2 thinkALS diagnostic guide for clinicians.
SOURCE: ALSA, 2021.

Management of ALS Symptoms

Approved medications for ALS (see Chapter 5) do not reverse the damage caused by the disease, but may slow progression of symptoms in some individuals. In addition to medications, treatment may include physical, occupational, speech, respiratory, and nutritional therapies. Heat or whirlpool therapy may help relieve muscle cramping, and exercise, in moderation, may help maintain muscle strength and function.

Most people with ALS eventually have trouble breathing as their diaphragm muscle and the muscles between their ribs that assist with air movement weaken. An individual's health care team will test their breathing regularly and, when necessary, provide mechanical ventilation to assist with breathing, overseen by a pulmonologist and respiratory therapist. In noninvasive ventilation, a small, portable machine delivers air through a face mask or nose insert, while invasive ventilation consists of a tube inserted permanently via surgery to create an opening in the trachea. The home health nurse and family caregivers receive instruction on cleaning and maintaining the tracheostomy tube and how to suction mucus.

Physical therapy can address pain, walking mobility, bracing, and equipment needs that can help a person living with ALS stay independent. Low-impact exercise can help maintain cardiovascular fitness, muscle strength, and range of motion for as long as possible. Regular exercise can also help improve a person's sense of well-being. Physical therapy can also include stretching, which can help prevent pain and muscle function.

Occupational therapy can help a person living with ALS find ways to remain independent despite hand, arm, and leg weakness. Adaptive equipment can help with performing activities of daily living, such as dressing, grooming, eating, and bathing, while braces, a walker, or wheelchair can make it easier for the person to move about without assistance. An occupational therapist can also suggest home modifications to make it easier and safer to move about in one's home.

Speech therapy can help a person living with ALS learn adaptive techniques to make their speech more understandable. Speech therapy can also help a person with ALS use other modes of communication, such as a smart phone app, alphabet board, or eye-tracking device. Speech therapists can record a person's voice for later use with a text-to-speech device if the individual can no longer speak clearly.

Nutritional support is important for ensuring that a person living with ALS is eating foods that are easier to swallow and meet their nutritional needs. Many people with ALS take nutritional supplements in the absence of effective medications.

Individuals living with ALS who receive care at an ALS multidisciplinary clinic may receive help from a social worker, who can assist with financial issues, insurance, acquiring needed DME, and getting outside financial assistance. Social workers and psychologists can also provide support for the person living with ALS and their family members.

Overlooked and Untreated Symptoms

Many secondary symptoms of ALS go unrecognized and untreated. Gastroparesis, or delayed emptying of the stomach, is an example of a common nonmotor ALS symptom that can cause severe discomfort (Toepfer et al.,

1999). Secondary complications related to immobility in ALS may also include deep venous thrombosis (DVT) and bedsores. The prevalence of these complications is not well known, although a recent study using an insurance claims database revealed that DVT occurs three times more frequently in persons with a diagnosis of ALS compared to controls without ALS (Kupelian et al., 2023).

Although people living with ALS experience many of these symptoms, they report that clinical care does not address them (Nicholson et al., 2018). In addition, clinical trials for therapeutic interventions may not capture data on ALS nonmotor symptoms, limiting understanding of the prevalence and potential effects of therapeutic agents (Goutman and Simmons, 2018). Researchers have proposed several possible reasons for the gap between high symptom prevalence and low rates of treatment, including a lack of high-quality evidence of effectiveness for interventions to treat secondary symptoms, lack of incentive for pharmaceutical companies to study off-label medications approved for more common diseases, and lack of training for neurologists in palliative care interventions (Goutman and Simmons, 2018).

Multidisciplinary Care

Chapter 4 describes in detail what research has found regarding how individuals living with ALS receive clinical care and the challenges facing the current care system. It also presents the committee's recommendations for creating a coordinated, sustainable ALS care and research system. In brief, there is a consensus in the field that a team of health care professionals in specialized ALS clinics should provide comprehensive care to an individual living with ALS. This model of multidisciplinary care includes a physician, physical therapist, occupational therapist, speech pathologist, dietitian, social worker, respiratory therapist, and nurse case manager (Miller et al., 2009b). Multidisciplinary care in an ALS specialty clinic is the standard of care for all individuals living with ALS, but access to such care is not universal (Galvin et al., 2017; Martin et al., 2017; Miller et al., 2009a; Pascual Martinez et al., 2019). According to ALSA, it is estimated that ALSA-certified multidisciplinary care clinics only serve a little more than 40 percent of individuals with ALS (ALSA, 2023). However, it is not known precisely how many of the approximately 30,000 individuals living with ALS are receiving care at an ALS clinic (ALSA, 2023; Galvin et al., 2017; Martin et al., 2017; Pascual Martinez et al., 2019).

RACIAL INEQUITIES IN ALS DIAGNOSIS, CARE, AND OUTCOMES

Race and ethnicity are associated with the risk of developing ALS, with non-Hispanic White individuals at substantially higher risk than non-Hispanic Black, Hispanic, and non-Hispanic individuals of other races and ethnicities (Roberts et al., 2016). The increased risk for non-Hispanic White individuals was only slightly attenuated when accounting for sex, socioeconomic status and health insurance, or place of birth. However, Hispanic and non-Hispanic Black individuals with ALS died at an earlier age than non-Hispanic White individuals with ALS (see Table 2-2).

Research has found there is a three-fold higher rate of tracheostomy and invasive ventilation and lower rates of noninvasive ventilation for Black individuals compared to White individuals living with ALS (Qadri et al., 2019). This may result from Black individuals living with ALS experiencing longer delays in receiving their diagnosis than White people living with ALS, which could lead to Black individuals living with ALS having lower baseline respiratory and functional status compared to White people living with ALS (Brand et al., 2021). While this may explain why Black individuals living with ALS have higher rates of tracheostomy and invasive ventilation, one study found that a greater percentage of people of color living with ALS chose tracheostomy over noninvasive ventilation compared to White people living with ALS (Brockenbrough et al., 2023).

One reason suggested for the delay in diagnosing ALS in Black individuals may be the result of some clinicians believing that Black people cannot develop certain diseases, including ALS (Carter, 2021). One study found that "Epistemological biases in scientific research, coupled with biases in public awareness systems, lead to inadequate consideration of who can or cannot contract certain diseases" and that "Gender and racial biases held by medical professional ALS community are written off as unknowns of disease etiology and pathology" (Carter, 2022). The author of that paper also made this comment:

> Despite [some] Black patients' learned mistrust of the medical system and often after multiple failed attempts to receive care or answers, ethnographic vignettes reveal that Black people with [ALS] and their caregivers continue to fight to be heard by the medical establishment. (Carter, 2022, p. 1)

In fact, multiple studies have documented that many physicians discount or disbelieve symptoms reported by Black individuals based on the long-discounted myth that there are innate racial differences between Black and White people's bodies (Hoffman et al., 2016; Hogarth, 2019; Oliver et al., 2014).

One study found that Black, Hispanic, and Asian individuals with ALS were more likely to die in an acute care facility versus at home or in hospice

TABLE 2-2 Adjusted Hazard Ratios (95% confidence intervals [CIs]) for Amyotrophic Lateral Sclerosis (ALS) Mortality by Race/Ethnicity, National Longitudinal Mortality Study, Women and Men Age 25 Years or Older, 1973–2011

	Participants		ALS deaths, n	Age at ALS death, y, mean (SD)	Model 1: Adjusted for sex, HR (95% CI)	Model 2: Further adjusted for socioeconomic status[a] and health insurance, HR (95% CI)	Model 3: Further adjusted for place of birth and presence of a Social Security number, HR (95% CI)
Race/ethnicity	No.	Person-years					
White, non-Hispanic	1,593,523	25,304,899	1,129	70.14 (10.98)	1.0 (Reference)	1.0 (Reference)	1.0 (Reference)
Black, non-Hispanic	200,280	2,805,086	62	64.63 (12.57)	0.58 (0.46–0.73)[b]	0.61 (0.48– 0.78)[b]	0.61 (0.48–0.78)[b]
Hispanic	216,922	2,819,176	54	68.73 (11.59)	0.56 (0.41–0.76)[b]	0.60 (0.44–0.82)[c]	0.64 (0.46–0.88)[c]
Other races, non-Hispanic	100,141	1,167,743	20	70.37 (13.00	0.46 (0.28–0.75)[c]	0.47 (0.29–0.76)[c]	0.52 (0.31–0.86)[d]
Missing	45,674	927,977	34	66.25 (10.49)	0.87 (0.62–1.20)	0.93 (0.67–1.29)	0.93 (0.67–1.29)

NOTES: [a] Socioeconomic status is measured by (1) income categorized in 5 levels, (2) household income as a percentage of the poverty line in 4 levels, (3) ownership or rental of home, and (4) educational attainment in 5 levels, all at time of survey.

[b] p<0.001.

[c] p<0.01.

[d] p<0.05.

CI = confidence interval; HR = hazards ratio; SD = standard deviation.

SOURCE: Roberts et al., 2016.

than White individuals with ALS (Goutman et al., 2014). Regarding this finding, the authors of this study stated:

> Although this may represent preferences such as the aggressiveness of care at end of life in these groups, this could be related to other factors including lack of access or affordability of home care services or availability of unpaid caregivers that prevent patients from staying at home at the end of life. (Goutman et al., 2014, p. 3)

This finding is important given that not dying at home is generally associated with not dying peacefully (Mandler et al., 2001). In addition, where someone dies has been proposed as a quality measure for end-of-life care for all diseases (Gruneir et al., 2007).

CONCLUDING COMMENTS

As outlined in the rest of this report, making ALS a livable disease will ultimately require many additional years of research. However, as this chapter makes clear, there are steps to take now toward this goal. Minimizing the many day-to-day challenges confronting people living with ALS, the difficulty obtaining the necessary care and services, the emotional and mental health toll of having a progressively disabling and invariably fatal disease, and the economic burden that can devastate a family's finances, would be a big step toward making ALS a livable disease.

Diagnostic delay is a major challenge the ALS clinical community must address to improve the duration and quality of life for individuals living with ALS. This will require better educating primary care physicians and general neurologists about this disease. In addition, there are many often overlooked secondary symptoms of ALS that require additional education among clinicians and attention in individuals living with ALS. Finally, guaranteeing equitable and affordable access to high-quality care for all individuals, regardless of socioeconomic status or geographic location, is essential to making ALS a livable disease.

REFERENCES

Alquati, S., L. Ghirotto, L. De Panfilis, C. Autelitano, E. Bertocchi, G. Artioli, F. Sireci, S. Tanzi, and S. Sacchi. 2022. Negotiating the beginning of care: A grounded theory study of health services for amyotrophic lateral sclerosis. *Brain Sci* 12(12).

ALSA (ALS Assocation). 2021. *thinkALS™ for faster diagnosis.* https://www.ALS.org/thinkALS (accessed April 3, 2024).

ALSA. 2023. *ALS around the globe: Improved access to ALS multidisciplinary care— the science of where.* https://www.als.org/blog/als-around-globe-improved-access-als-multidisciplinary-care-science-where (accessed April 3, 2024).

Babu, S., N. M. Thakur, R. S. Bedlack, Z. Simmons, and L. Falivena. 2022. Early diagnosis and the need for novel therapeutics in ALS: Highlights from a recent symposium. Medscape, Virtual.

Brand, D., M. Polak, J. D. Glass, and C. N. Fournier. 2021. Comparison of phenotypic characteristics and prognosis between Black and White patients in a tertiary ALS clinic. *Neurology* 96(6):e840–e844.

Brockenbrough, P., D. Carter, Q. Fan, M. Gebhardt, A. Shields, and K. Gwathmey. 2023. *Retrospective analysis of the racial diversity in invasive ventilation decisions by patients with ALS.* Paper presented at 22nd Annual Meeting of the Northeast ALS Consortium, Clearwater, FL.

Carter, C. 2021. *The racial thinking behind ALS diagnosis.* https://www.anthropology-news.org/articles/the-racial-thinking-behind-ALS-diagnosis/?utm_source=rss&utm_medium=rss&utm_campaign=the-racial-thinking-behind-ALS-diagnosis#citation (accessed April 2, 2024).

Carter, C. R. 2022. Gaslighting: ALS, anti-blackness, and medicine. *Feminist Anthropology* 3(2):235–245.

Choi, B. C., and A. W. Pak. 2006. Multidisciplinarity, interdisciplinarity and transdisciplinarity in health research, services, education and policy: 1. Definitions, objectives, and evidence of effectiveness. *Clin Invest Med* 29(6):351–364.

de Almeida, F. E. O., A. K. do Carmo Santana, and F. O. de Carvalho. 2021. Multidisciplinary care in amyotrophic lateral sclerosis: A systematic review and meta-analysis. *Neurol Sci* 42(3):911–923.

Falcão de Campos, C., M. Gromicho, H. Uysal, J. Grosskreutz, M. Kuzma-Kozakiewicz, M. Oliveira Santos, S. Pinto, S. Petri, M. Swash, and M. de Carvalho. 2021. Delayed diagnosis and diagnostic pathway of ALS patients in Portugal: Where can we improve? *Front Neurol* 12:761355.

Falcão de Campos, C., M. Gromicho, H. Uysal, J. Grosskreutz, M. Kuzma-Kozakiewicz, M. Oliveira Santos, S. Pinto, S. Petri, M. Swash, and M. de Carvalho. 2022. Trends in the diagnostic delay and pathway for amyotrophic lateral sclerosis patients across different countries. *Front Neurol* 13:1064619.

Galvin, M., C. Madden, S. Maguire, M. Heverin, A. Vajda, A. Staines, and O. Hardiman. 2015. Patient journey to a specialist amyotrophic lateral sclerosis multidisciplinary clinic: An exploratory study. *BMC Health Services Research* 15:571.

Galvin, M., P. Ryan, S. Maguire, M. Heverin, C. Madden, A. Vajda, C. Normand, and O. Hardiman. 2017. The path to specialist multidisciplinary care in amyotrophic lateral sclerosis: A population-based study of consultations, interventions and costs. *PLOS One* 12(6):e0179796.

Goutman, S. A., and Z. Simmons. 2018. Symptom management in amyotrophic lateral sclerosis: We can do better. *Muscle Nerve* 57(1):1–3.

Goutman, S. A., D. G. Nowacek, J. F. Burke, K. A. Kerber, L. E. Skolarus, and B. C. Callaghan. 2014. Minorities, men, and unmarried amyotrophic lateral sclerosis patients are more likely to die in an acute care facility. *Amyotroph Lateral Scler Frontotemporal Degener* 15(5–6):440–443.

Gruneir, A., V. Mor, S. Weitzen, R. Truchil, J. Teno, and J. Roy. 2007. Where people die: A multilevel approach to understanding influences on site of death in America. *Med Care Res Rev* 64(4):351–378.

Gwathmey, K. G., P. Corcia, C. J. McDermott, A. Genge, S. Sennfält, M. de Carvalho, and C. Ingre. 2023. Diagnostic delay in amyotrophic lateral sclerosis. *Euro J Neurol* 30(9):2595–2601.

Hoffman, K. M., S. Trawalter, J. R. Axt, and M. N. Oliver. 2016. Racial bias in pain assessment and treatment recommendations, and false beliefs about biological differences between Blacks and Whites. *Proceedings of the National Academy of Sciences of the United States of America* 113(16):4296–4301.

Hogarth, R. A. 2019. The myth of innate racial differences between White and Black people's bodies: Lessons from the 1793 yellow fever epidemic in Philadelphia, Pennsylvania. *American Journal of Public Health* 109(10):1339–1341.

Hogden, A., G. Foley, R. D. Henderson, N. James, and S. M. Aoun. 2017. Amyotrophic lateral sclerosis: Improving care with a multidisciplinary approach. *J Multidisciplin Healthcare* 10:205–215.

Kraemer, M., M. Buerger, and P. Berlit. 2010. Diagnostic problems and delay of diagnosis in amyotrophic lateral sclerosis. *Clin Neurol Neurosurg* 112(2):103–105.

Kupelian, V., E. Viscidi, S. Hall, L. Li, S. Eaton, A. Dilley, N. Currier, T. Ferguson, and L. Fanning. 2023. Increased risk of venous thromboembolism in patients with amyotrophic lateral sclerosis: Results from a US insurance claims database study. *Neurol Clin Pract* 13(1):e200110.

Ludolph, A., L. Dupuis, E. Kasarskis, F. Steyn, S. Ngo, and C. McDermott. 2023. Nutritional and metabolic factors in amyotrophic lateral sclerosis. *Nat Rev Neurol* 19(9):511–524.

Mandler, R. N., F. A. Anderson, Jr., R. G. Miller, L. Clawson, M. Cudkowicz, and M. Del Bene. 2001. The ALS patient care database: Insights into end-of-life care in ALS. *Amyotroph Lateral Scler Other Motor Neuron Dis* 2(4):203–208.

Martin, S., E. Trevor-Jones, S. Khan, K. Shaw, D. Marchment, A. Kulka, C. E. Ellis, R. Burman, M. R. Turner, L. Carroll, L. Mursaleen, P. N. Leigh, C. E. Shaw, N. Pearce, D. Stahl, and A. Al-Chalabi. 2017. The benefit of evolving multidisciplinary care in ALS: A diagnostic cohort survival comparison. *Amyotroph Lateral Scler Frontotemp Degener* 18(7–8):569–575.

Matharan, M., S. Mathis, S. Bonabaud, L. Carla, A. Soulages, and G. Le Masson. 2020. Minimizing the diagnostic delay in amyotrophic lateral sclerosis: The role of nonneurologist practitioners. *Neurol Res Inter* 2020:1473981.

MDA (Muscular Dystrophy Association). 2018. *Highlights of the MDA U.S. Neuromuscular Disease Registry (2013–2016).* https://www.mda.org/sites/default/files/MDA-Registry-Report-Highlights-Digital_9-2018.pdf (accessed May 16, 2024).

Miller, R. G., C. E. Jackson, E. J. Kasarskis, J. D. England, D. Forshew, W. Johnston, S. Kalra, J. S. Katz, H. Mitsumoto, J. Rosenfeld, C. Shoesmith, M. J. Strong, and S. C. Woolley. 2009a. Practice parameter update: The care of the patient with amyotrophic lateral sclerosis: Drug, nutritional, and respiratory therapies (an evidence-based review). Report of the Quality Standards Subcommittee of the American Academy of Neurology. *Neurology* 73(15):1218–1226.

Miller, R. G., C. E. Jackson, E. J. Kasarskis, J. D. England, D. Forshew, W. Johnston, S. Kalra, J. S. Katz, H. Mitsumoto, J. Rosenfeld, C. Shoesmith, M. J. Strong, and S. C. Woolley. 2009b. Practice parameter update: The care of the patient with amyotrophic lateral sclerosis: Multidisciplinary care, symptom management, and cognitive/behavioral impairment (an evidence-based review). Report of the Quality Standards Subcommittee of the American Academy of Neurology. *Neurology* 73(15):1227–1233.

Ng, L., F. Khan, and S. Mathers. 2009. Multidisciplinary care for adults with amyotrophic lateral sclerosis or motor neuron disease. *Cochrane Database of System Rev* (4):CD007425.

Nicholson, K., A. Murphy, E. McDonnell, J. Shapiro, E. Simpson, J. Glass, H. Mitsumoto, D. Forshew, R. Miller, and N. Atassi. 2018. Improving symptom management for people with amyotrophic lateral sclerosis. *Muscle Nerve* 57(1):20–24.

Oliver, M. N., K. M. Wells, J. A. Joy-Gaba, C. B. Hawkins, and B. A. Nosek. 2014. Do physicians' implicit views of African Americans affect clinical decision making? *J Am Board Fam Med* 27(2):177–188.

Paganoni, S., E. A. Macklin, A. Lee, A. Murphy, J. Chang, A. Zipf, M. Cudkowicz, and N. Atassi. 2014. Diagnostic timelines and delays in diagnosing amyotrophic lateral sclerosis (ALS). *Amyotroph Lateral Scler Frontotemp Degener* 15(5–6):453–456.

Pascual Martinez, N., S. Martín Bote, E. Martínez Repiso, T. Gómez Caravaca, L. Muñoz Cabello, C. Gómez Rebollo, M. Mejías Ruiz, M. Fernández Alcaide, A. L. Luna Jiménez, M. J. Toril Redondo, J. M. Martín Muñoz, M. Posadas De Julián, M. J. González Benítez, R. Gómez Gómez, and M. L. Raya Seco De Herrera. 2019. The benefit of multidisciplinary care in ALS. *Euro Respirat J* 54(Suppl 63):PA4028.

Qadri, S., C. D. Langefeld, C. Milligan, J. B. Caress, and M. S. Cartwright. 2019. Racial differences in intervention rates in individuals with ALS. *Neurology* 92(17):e1969.

Richards, D., J. A. Morren, and E. P. Pioro. 2021. Time to diagnosis and factors affecting diagnostic delay in amyotrophic lateral sclerosis. In *Amyotrophic lateral sclerosis*, edited by T. Araki. Brisbane, Australia: Exon Publications.

Roberts, A. L., N. J. Johnson, J. T. Chen, M. E. Cudkowicz, and M. G. Weisskopf. 2016. Race/ethnicity, socioeconomic status, and ALS mortality in the United States. *Neurology* 87(22):2300–2308.

Rosa Silva, J. P., J. B. Santiago Júnior, E. L. dos Santos, F. O. de Carvalho, I. M. P. de França Costa, and D. M. F. d. Mendonça. 2020. Quality of life and functional independence in amyotrophic lateral sclerosis: A systematic review. *Neurosci Biobehav Rev* 111:1–11.

Takei, K., T. Kikumi, F. Takahashi, M. Hirai, and J. Palumbo. 2017. An assessment of treatment guidelines, clinical practices, demographics, and progression of disease among patients with amyotrophic lateral sclerosis in Japan, the United States, and Europe. *Amyotrophic Lateral Sclerosis and Frontotemporal Degeneration* 18:88–97.

Toepfer, M., C. Folwaczny, H. Lochmuller, M. Schroeder, R. L. Riepl, D. Pongratz, and W. Muller-Felber. 1999. Noninvasive (13)c-octanoic acid breath test shows delayed gastric emptying in patients with amyotrophic lateral sclerosis. *Digestion* 60(6):567–571.

Williams, J. R., D. Fitzhenry, L. Grant, D. Martyn, and D. A. Kerr. 2013. Diagnosis pathway for patients with amyotrophic lateral sclerosis: Retrospective analysis of the US Medicare longitudinal claims database. *BMC Neurology* 13(1):160.

Witzel, S., M. Wagner, C. Zhao, K. Kandler, E. Graf, R. Berutti, K. Oexle, D. Brenner, J. Winkelmann, and A. C. Ludolph. 2022. Fast versus slow disease progression in amyotrophic lateral sclerosis–clinical and genetic factors at the edges of the survival spectrum. *Neurobiol Aging* 119:117–126.

Wu, J. M., M. T. Tam, K. Buch, F. Khairati, L. Wilson, E. Bannerman, A. Guerrero, A. Eisen, W. Toyer, T. Stevenson, and J. M. Robillard. 2022. The impact of respite care from the perspectives and experiences of people with amyotrophic lateral sclerosis and their care partners: A qualitative study. *BMC Palliat Care* 21(1):26.

Yersak, J., S. Birhane, T. Heiman-Patterson, C. Lomen-Hoerth, B. Oskarsson, and S. Babu. 2021. Cms-03 thinkALS: A user-friendly and comprehensive ALS diagnosis and referal tool for general neurologists. *Amyotroph Lateral Scler Frontotemp Degener* 22:202–233.

3

Making ALS Livable in the Near Term

ABSTRACT

As part of its charge, the committee was asked to recommend key actions for the public, private, and nonprofit sectors to undertake to make amyotrophic lateral sclerosis (ALS) a livable disease within a decade. In Chapter 4, the committee makes recommendations that, if implemented, would create an accessible, coordinated, and sustainable ALS care and research system. While these long-term actions are critical to improving ALS research and care for future people with ALS, the committee recognized the acute need and opportunity for immediate, short-term actions that would make ALS a more livable disease today. This chapter provides the evidence and supporting rationale for recommended actions that, if implemented immediately, would achieve that goal.

INSURANCE CHALLENGES

The other insurance companies didn't do very much. Doctors saw me and wanted to check my muscles and that was it. Anything I needed I had to pay for. When they told me I needed a power chair, the first one I got I had to help pay for that, and you know how much they cost.
—*Jim Clingman, person living with ALS*

One the most vexing problems individuals living with ALS and their caregivers face is negotiating with insurance companies to obtain the services they need. To start, most insurance coverage policies do not easily accommodate the unique needs of an individual living with ALS, which

67

can lead to stressful, frustrating interactions with an insurer. As the ALS Association (ALSA) notes in its advice to people living with ALS and their caregivers, insurance is not the easiest subject for anyone to understand because of its complexity, whether it is premiums, deductibles, out-of-pocket maximum payments, and pharmacy coverage based on tier medication systems, just to name a few. According to the ALS Association, "many people do not even know where to start or what questions to ask" when dealing with an insurer due to the complexities of the system, as well as their unique needs (ALSA, 2023a).

Social Security Disability Insurance and Medicare

Persons with ALS experience a variety of insurance situations that depend on a number of factors, including whether a person is still working and if an individual is eligible to receive Social Security Disability Insurance (SSDI). Individuals who have worked for a minimum period in jobs covered by Social Security and have a qualifying condition, such as ALS, are eligible for SSDI. Once a person with ALS receives SSDI, which includes a monthly payment, they also become eligible for Medicare, which provides medical care and equipment.

The federal Medicare program, administered by the Centers for Medicare & Medicaid Services (CMS), is offered to individuals aged 65 and above. However, there are two exceptions to the age 65 requirement: individuals with end-stage renal disease or a disability have access to Medicare coverage. Because ALS causes disability, persons with ALS under age 65 qualify for Medicare. In addition, persons with ALS are exempt from the usual waiting period before Medicare coverage can begin and therefore can receive benefits the first month they are eligible. Many people with ALS receive SSDI and Medicare, but not everyone will be eligible based on their work history. In particular, a younger person diagnosed with ALS with limited work history may not meet the required work history to receive disability benefits and Medicare.

There is uncertainty as to the number of persons living with ALS who do not have access to SSDI and Medicare given their work history. In addition, some people with ALS are not even aware of the benefits they are eligible to receive through SSDI and Medicare. Congress has recognized that ALS is an exceptional disease and corrected eligibility requirements for federal programs to ensure persons with ALS receive access without delay (Korbey, 2023).

For people with ALS who are still working, unique challenges may emerge. SSDI applicants are not allowed to earn more than a certain amount per month, so earning too much through their work could disqualify them from receiving disability benefits. For a person with ALS who is able to continue working, this may leave considerable gaps in access to disability-related services and financial strain.

For example, a person with ALS, Bruce Rosenblum, who continued working well into his disease course and died in December 2023, described his situation:

> Insurance coverage for caregiving is inadequate for ALS patients on disability and virtually nonexistent for patients like myself who, although disabled, are not on disability. Three years ago, my wife retired to become my primary caregiver. But serving as the primary caregiver for a spouse who is progressing through ALS is a physically and emotionally draining job for which additional support is necessary. We supplement my wife's care, when we are able to find caregivers, which is an entirely separate challenge, with 5 hours of professional caregiving coverage each morning to help with the most challenging activities of daily living. Thirty hours of weekly paid caregiving, which we have to pay for out of pocket, exceeded 50 percent of my take-home pay each of the last 3 years. Add together all of the other uncovered costs of ALS, and that has left us drawing on our retirement savings for most nonmedical living expenses.

The committee finds that even though Congress has recognized the exceptional nature of ALS and made important changes to eligibility requirements for federal programs to make it easier for people with ALS, not everyone with an ALS diagnosis is eligible to receive SSDI and access to Medicare. There is an opportunity to expand the status of ALS as a qualifying condition for Medicare coverage, such that persons with ALS are eligible for Medicare coverage regardless of employment history or other criteria influencing Medicare or SSDI eligibility.

Prior Authorization, Insurance Denials, and Appeals

People living with ALS can face challenges in acquiring medically indicated equipment, technology, and therapeutics and dealing with an often-convoluted system for obtaining prior authorizations. Prior authorization refers to a process in which insurance companies require a clinician or other qualified health professional to seek advance approval before providing certain services, tests, medications, equipment, or procedures. Prior authorization is a tool insurers use frequently as a means of controlling costs and avoiding unnecessary care. The committee was unable to find publicly available information or evidence as to whether prior authorization processes reduce unnecessary costs in ALS care, nor was the committee able to determine whether all prior authorization request denials for ALS are inappropriate. Frustration with prior authorization processes is also not unique to ALS—reforming prior authorization processes across the insurance industry are the focus of national efforts and are not restricted to just one disease area (AMA, 2022). CMS issued a final rule in January 2024 that requires payers to streamline prior authorization processes electronically and provide more information to patients about prior authorization processes including approvals, denials, or requests for more information beginning in January 2026. The new rule also requires payers to send prior authorization decisions within 72 hours for expedited or urgent requests and 7 calendar days for standard or nonurgent requests and publicly report certain prior authorization metrics annually.[1] Prior authorization challenges are largely associated with Medicare Advantage plans and not traditional Medicare.

Insurance companies and Medicare Advantage plans may deny a prior authorization request and require an individual to "fail first," which means they will only give authorization if the individual first tries and fails a treatment or is not well served by a piece of equipment. ALSA has reported many examples of Medicare Advantage plans and other private insurers denying access to home mechanical ventilation (ALSA, 2024) despite evidence supporting the use of such equipment in reducing morbidity and mortality. For example, a clinician might order a specific ventilator for an individual living with ALS to use at home, and instead of approving the ventilator requested by the clinician, the insurance company might require that the individual first use and fail on a less expensive ventilator designed for chronic obstructive pulmonary disease patients to use. Importantly, less expensive ventilator devices often have inadequate battery capabilities thereby limiting mobility for people living with ALS and further impairing quality of life. Again, there is an absence of publicly available data from insurance companies showing that prior authorization processes reduce costs while improving outcomes for individuals living with ALS. The committee would find it unacceptable for a person diagnosed with ALS to be forced to use a ventilator that provides less effective breathing support for ALS because it is designed for another type of disease. Cost-controlling measures are only appropriate when two devices are equivalent and deliver similar results and value to a patient.

A 2022 ALSA survey of people living with ALS and caregivers found that one in three people who submitted a prior authorization request or claim were denied at least once (ALSA, 2023b). The top five denials were for prescription medications or medication delivery supplies; wheelchair accessories; power wheelchairs; in-home physical, occupational, or speech therapy; and a wheelchair-accessible vehicle or vehicle modifications.

After receiving an insurance denial, an individual can make multiple appeals to the insurance company, the relevant state agency that regulates insurance companies in their state, and even contact journalists or the

---

[1]See CMS Interoperability and Prior Authorization final rule, CMS-0057-F.

media regarding denials of care, services, or equipment the individual deems necessary. According to an ALSA survey, 67 percent of those denied prior authorization and 47 percent who had a claim denied appealed the insurers decisions (ALSA, 2023b). The ALSA survey also found that participants had to appeal up to three times and wait up to 6 months for a resolution to their appeal, with approximately one-third of the appeals denied or only partially granted. Those individuals denied authorization or reimbursement had to either pay out of pocket; forgo the requested drug, service, or device; or discontinue care. The committee finds this length of delay unacceptable given the rapid disease course of ALS.

People responding to the ALSA survey reported frustration with Medicare denials and appeals. Often, individuals must first obtain the services or items in question and assume the financial risk before they can file an appeal (Center for Medicare Advocacy, 2016).

The most common reason for the denial of a claim involves the determination of whether there is medical necessity. Sometimes, a medication or procedure that a care provider deems important is not seen this way by an insurance company. When this occurs, a care provider may need to show proof of the value of a particular treatment over alternatives. Some Medicare contractors issue denials because they mistakenly believe that Medicare only covers skilled services such as physical, speech, and occupational therapy when those services will lead to an improvement in symptoms (Center for Medicare Advocacy, 2018).

The committee finds that ALS is a heterogeneous, multisystem disease that requires a proactive and anticipatory approach to care. Prior authorization processes can be inappropriately blunt tools used by insurers for many services, procedures, tests, and medications that individuals living with ALS need to improve their quality of life. Lengthy prior authorization processes rob an individual living with ALS of their most precious resource—time. Prior authorization processes also add strain and sap energy from clinical staff. There is a need for prior authorization processes to be streamlined, expedited, or removed for ALS care given the time course of the disease.

INADEQUATE HOME SERVICES

I had physical therapy in my home. I have to go through my primary care provider to get the prescription to submit to the company. Everything takes a long time to get approved or how many visits get approved, which to me seems very strange. It's almost like I have to go back to my primary care provider every once in a while to say, "Hey, I still have ALS." Why do we have to waste time going over something like this? It's not like ALS goes away. Now I pay out of pocket for the physical therapy because the insurance is just a pain to get it covered. To me, it is so important for me because during that physical therapy is probably the only time where I feel less pain in my joints and everywhere. It gives me a physical break but also an emotional support system where afterward emotionally I have the capability to be more interactive with my son, for example, and do things together.

—Julian Rodriguez, person living with ALS,
as described to the committee during August 2023 public workshop

I require a home health aide 12 hours a day, 7 days a week. My mother is a huge part of my care team. She makes me healthy food and cooks for my husband and my daughter. She covers when aides are not available for work.

—Desiree Galvez Kessler, person living with ALS,
as described to the committee during August 2023 public workshop

People with ALS need significant supports at home to maintain quality of life. The symptoms of ALS impede basic motor function and day-to-day activities. Living with ALS means continually adapting one's living environment to meet changing needs as the disease progresses. Home health care may be an early need for people living with ALS with rapid progression or co-occurring frontotemporal dementia.

Home health care can include assistance from home health aides with activities of daily living; physical, occupational, and speech therapy; respiratory care and ventilator management; complex nursing care; and hospice. Privately hired caregivers or home health care agencies may provide care in the home; the latter are bound by licensure statutes and state and federal regulations regarding care staff competency. Home health care agencies may also be accredited, such as by the Community Health Accreditation Partner, and certified by CMS.

There are four main challenges persons living with ALS face to receive adequate home health care: choosing a home health care provider, being accepted by a home health care provider, paying for home health care, and coordinating home health care with the medical care team. Several organizations, including ALSA,[2] AARP,[3] I AM ALS,[4] and CMS,[5] have prepared guides to help individuals living with ALS and their families choose a home health care provider.

Hiring a home health care agency is expensive, and an individual's insurance may not cover all services. CMS does not have the authority to pay for concomitant services at home and as an outpatient,[6] leaving some individuals with ALS challenged to receive needed care in the clinic and also at home.

---

[2]Available at http://www.alsa.org/als-care/resources/fyi/choosing-a-home-health-care.html (accessed May 10, 2024).

[3]Available at https://assets.aarp.org/external_sites/caregiving/checklists/checklist_inHomeCare.html (accessed May 10, 2024).

[4]Available at https://www.iamals.org/wp-content/uploads/2020/10/Questions-to-Ask-a-Potential-Home-Health-Agency.pdf (accessed May 10, 2024).

[5]Available at https://www.cms.gov/Medicare/Quality-Initiatives-Patient-Assessment-Instruments/HomeHealthQualityInits/Downloads/HHQIHHBenefits.pdf (accessed May 10, 2024).

[6]42 USC 1395fff.

Medicare certified home health care is unlimited in duration and coverage continues to be available so long as skilled care is needed and threshold criteria are met. Intermittent care refers to noncoverage of daily skilled care after 21 days.[7] To be eligible for any home health care support, individuals must have a formal ALS diagnosis and be certified by their doctor as being unable to leave their home without considerable effort and assistance.

For individuals meeting low-income requirements, Medicaid can supplement Medicare. While each state sets its own policies, most state Medicaid plans will pay for personal care services, in addition to skilled care services. Some states also offer "waivers" to keep people out of long-term care facilities and in their homes for as long as possible, since the latter is more cost-efficient.

Some private insurance plans cover private duty nursing and home care expenses for people living with ALS. Long-term care insurance—if the policy covers ALS—will pay for in-home skilled nursing, therapeutic care, and personal care. There are also many organizations and local foundations that help pay for home health care for individuals with ALS.

Good coordination between a home care provider and an individual's clinical team can benefit patients, family caregivers, providers, and payer organizations by reducing hospital admissions and emergency department visits and lowering health care costs (Friedman et al., 2016; Möckli et al., 2021). Medicare's Conditions of Participation,[8] which a home health agency must satisfy to participate in Medicare and Medicaid programs, includes care coordination requirements.

Conclusive, nationwide data on use, access, and experiences with home health services for Medicare beneficiaries living with ALS is limited. There are approximately 66 million Medicare beneficiaries, and even if every one of the approximately 30,000 people living with ALS in the United States were enrolled in Medicare, less than half of 1 percent of Medicare beneficiaries will have ALS at any given time. Medicare use data by disease category is not readily available, particularly for rare diseases such as ALS. However, recent CMS data reveal a worrisome, continuous downward trend in Medicare home health use and declines in skilled nursing, physical therapy, occupational therapy, and speech therapy (AARP, 2023). Because of a lack of CMS analysis of these data, it is unknown why these trends are emerging and whether the appropriate level of home health care is being provided to Medicare beneficiaries (AARP, 2023).

Some home health care agencies wrongly deny that Medicare will pay for their services (Center for Medicare Advocacy, 2013). Medicare policies and

---

[7]Intermittent skilled nursing care is care that is needed or given on fewer than 7 days a week (i.e., not daily) or (daily) less than 8 hours a day over a period of 21 days or less.

[8]Available at https://www.federalregister.gov/documents/2017/01/13/2017-00283/medicare-and-medicaid-program-conditions-of-participation-for-home-health-agencies (accessed May 10, 2024).

incentives generally favor short-term improvement goals, such as posthospital patients who improve, even though Medicare home health coverage is not limited in time for those who meet threshold criteria, nor is restoration or improvements of one's condition required.

The limitations in access to high-quality, affordable home health care that exist in the United States have a significant effect on the ability of unpaid caregivers to provide the necessary care for their loved ones with ALS. A 2023 scoping review found persistent unmet needs for caregivers in the following areas: emotional and psychological needs; assistive devices and technology; information and education; and human and professional resources and services (Young et al., 2023). Despite the predictable trajectory of ALS, the biopsychosocial and equipment interventions available for people living with ALS were generally not provided proactively. The authors suggest that home health care for people with ALS and the experience of their caregivers should be addressed by examining these areas of need: interdisciplinary care, including home-health and end-of-life care; caregiver outcomes including burnout; durable medical equipment (DME) and technology; patients' and caregivers' diverse racial, cultural, and social backgrounds; and policy implications. Young et al. stated a goal to work with the American Academy of Neuromuscular and Electrodiagnostic Medicine to convene an expert panel to develop consensus-based ALS home health medical standards. The guidelines would exist to promote greater accessibility to needed services and supports.

The committee found that precise data are lacking around home health care use for individuals living with ALS who are Medicare beneficiaries. National trends in home health care use and the experiences of individuals living with ALS shared with this committee indicate there is a serious challenge in accessing high-quality, affordable home health care for the complex and evolving needs of people living with ALS. Many individuals living with ALS are not able to get legally covered care and services.

HIGH OUT-OF-POCKET COSTS

The financial side of it has been very frustrating and difficult but it is also time-consuming, and I feel like time is the biggest, most important currency that we live with. If something takes a couple months to get in, in just a couple of months my body may change, and the reasons why we got those adjustments in the first place may not be suitable now.

—*Julian Rodriguez, person living with ALS*

My parents spent well over $100,000.00 on costs related to my mom's ALS even though she only survived 16 months after diagnosis. Compassion Care ALS helped my family a lot with many of these incidental things such as wheelchair-accessible van rentals when needed.

—*Jean Swidler, presymptomatic genetic carrier and caregiver,*
Executive Director of Genetic ALS & FTD: End the Legacy

The looming fear of financial catastrophe can have a negative impact on a person with ALS and their current quality of life. The total cost of ALS care, including costs paid by insurers, is higher than it is for other neurological diseases (Gladman and Zinman, 2015). A systematic review of 12 studies from eight countries published between 2001 and 2015 indicated the total annual cost per person living with ALS in the United States was approximately $70,000; the United States had the highest total costs of those countries in the review (Gladman and Zinman, 2015). One case study of a single person with ALS found that from 2000 to 2010, their total cost of care was more than $1.4 million in 2013 USD (Obermann and Lyon, 2015). Given inflation, recent ALS drug approvals, including Relyvrio,[9] which costs $158,000 per year for an individual patient, and an overall increase in technology options (e.g., communication devices), the committee surmises that the total annual cost of ALS care is far higher than estimates based on data from 2000 to 2015. While understanding the total economic impact of ALS on individuals, insurers, and governments can be useful, understanding the out-of-pocket costs individuals and families affected by ALS are experiencing, including lost wages, is also critical to understanding the true financial impact of the disease.

ALS was the most common neurological condition that users created campaigns for on GoFundMe, a crowdsourced fundraising platform, between 2011 and 2021 (Galvin et al., 2023). People with ALS and their families often seek financial support for home modifications or services and devices they need to make the disease more livable. Regardless of condition, most individuals seeking financial assistance through crowdfunding had insurance, highlighting the financial burdens faced by individuals living with ALS and their families resulting from inadequate insurance support.

The committee received perspectives from several individuals living with ALS and their family members regarding the amount they spend out of pocket to cover care and services that insurance did not cover or denied. Here is a description of some of those experiences:

- Bruce Rosenblum, an individual with lived ALS experience who participated in the committee's August 2023 workshop and died in December 2023, spent more than 50 percent of his take-home pay over the last 3 years on 30 hours per week of professional caregiving to help each weekday morning with the more challenging activities of daily living. Bruce's wife retired 3 years earlier to become his primary caregiver but, as the committee also heard from other individuals living with ALS, additional assistance in

---

[9]As the committee was finishing its work on this report, the company developing AMX0035/Relyvrio announced the latest results of a Phase 3 trial in which the drug performed no better than placebo and the company began the process of removing the drug from the market.

the home is needed. Bruce also paid $5,000 out-of-pocket for a fully electric hospital bed and a low air mattress. Insurance denied coverage for these items, though they were necessary because his wife and primary caregiver lives with a muscle condition and could not reasonably care for him using the less effective items insurance would approve—a semielectric hospital bed and a manual Hoyer lift.

- Committee member Mindy Uhrlaub reported her mother paid $25,000 for a power wheelchair Medicare did not cover.
- Ady Barkan, a person with ALS who died in November 2023, spent $40,000 per month for 24-hour care that was reimbursed primarily through insurance via an ad hoc arrangement (King, 2024).

Of those individuals who responded to an ALSA survey on mobility challenges, 26 percent reported they paid at least some of the out-of-pocket costs for a power wheelchair and 47 percent said insurers refused to pay for their power wheelchair seat elevation (ALSA, 2021) (see Figure 3-1). A recently updated CMS policy now covers seat elevation systems for power wheelchairs (CMS, 2023a).

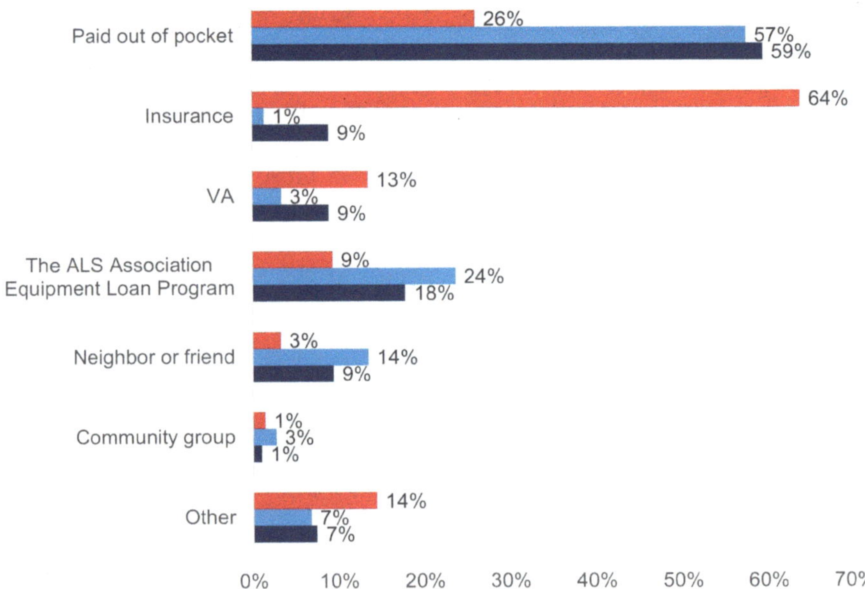

FIGURE 3-1 How individuals living with ALS pay for their mobility equipment. NOTE: Red bars = power wheelchair; light blue bars = portable ramp; dark blue bars = rollator.
SOURCE: ALSA, 2021.

Some individuals living with ALS also pay for traveling to participate in a clinical trial. A recent cost estimate of clinical trial participation comes from committee members affected by ALS. Joel Shamaskin, committee member and person living with ALS, participated in research at two study sites between 2016 and 2019 and paid $3,500 out of pocket to cover transportation, lodging, and meals associated with his research participation. Mindy Uhrlaub, committee member and at-risk ALS genetic carrier, spent more than $12,000 over the course of 2 years to support travel and accommodations associated with participating in longitudinal, observational research studies involving genetic carriers. These observational studies provided no compensation for participants, nor were participants able to benefit from taking an experimental drug in the context of a clinical trial. Out-of-pocket costs to participate in research are deterrents to participation, and the committee believes the appropriate budget for a clinical trial would anticipate and cover the costs associated with a person with ALS participating (Gelinas et al., 2018).

Drug Costs

Drug pricing policies and insurance decisions regarding whether to pay for a drug are complex and not fully transparent. As more ALS drugs are expected to achieve regulatory approval in the next decade, the pharmaceutical choices to treat this disease will grow, along with the costs to patients. While Chapter 5 discusses some of the trade-offs in drug development and approval decisions, there are also near-term opportunities for reducing the out-of-pocket costs borne by people with ALS for drugs. The committee believes one opportunity to address the high cost of drugs to treat ALS is to negotiate drug prices.

As part of the Inflation Reduction Act of 2022, the Secretary of the U.S. Department of Health and Human Services is required to negotiate prices with drug companies for a small number of single-source, brand-name drugs or biologics without generic or biosimilar competitors covered by Medicare (Cubanski et al., 2023). To qualify for this negotiation, the drug must cost Medicare more than $200 million per year, cannot have a generic competitor, and cannot have a single orphan designation. While it is unlikely ALS drugs will qualify for negotiation under the Inflation Reduction Act criteria in the near future, other opportunities to negotiate the price of ALS drugs could positively affect people with ALS in terms of access to affordable drugs that would make the disease more livable.

ALS Organizations Assisting People with ALS

In addition to high out-of-pocket costs for care, equipment, and therapeutics, there are other direct costs that individuals living with ALS and their families bear. Some persons with ALS will have to move to a more accessible home, make significant home modifications that can cost tens of thousands of dollars, or purchase a wheelchair-accessible van, which can cost upward of $100,000. They may also have to pay for at-home care out of pocket. In addition, there is the loss of income that comes when the individual living with ALS can no longer work or when other adults in the household have to reduce their hours or forgo their job entirely to care for their loved one.

ALS organizations and patient-serving groups offer many different types of resources and sometimes direct financial assistance with home modifications or procuring a wheelchair-accessible van. However, access to these resources is fragmented and depends on where the person with ALS lives. For example, an ALSA chapter in Minnesota might offer assistance with home modification, but a chapter in another state will not. Each ALS organization, and sometimes each chapter within an organization, will have a different philanthropic model, area of focus, and resources. New organizations spun off of state and local ALSA chapters, such as ALS United, will likely result in more variation across the organizational landscape addressing ALS needs. While this structure means that not every ALS organization will be able to offer the same levels of support, an opportunity exists to coordinate and streamline information and resources so that a person with ALS and their family can receive the support they need. The committee heard from individuals with ALS lived experience—persons with ALS, current and former caregivers, and individuals at risk of developing ALS—that the fragmented nature of information and resources across 50-plus ALS organizations can be confusing to navigate, take significant effort and time, and contribute to overall stress and anxiety.

> As all of us know, this is an extremely expensive disease, not just in terms of the medicine but also in terms of all the support that you need, and so it was really important that I maintained a full-time role so that we could take some of that pressure off us as a family unit.
> —*Siobhan Pandya, former caregiver of a person living with ALS*

> At 45, my husband and I are supposed to be in the prime earning period of our lives, but he has not been able to work full-time due to having to care for me and our kids. I have had to drastically reduce my hours to 35 percent due to time and energy considerations and my inability to teach anymore. While I receive a disability check from my pension system, it doesn't add up to what we could be earning as a couple if I were healthy.
> —*Kristin Rankin, person living with ALS*

Recommendation 3-1: Facilitate expedited access to and coverage of essential ALS medical and support services.

The Centers for Medicare and Medicaid Services (CMS) and private insurers should act quickly to enable expedited access to the following essential ALS medical and support services:

a. Provide coverage for home based and outpatient physical and other support services for persons with ALS as necessary, of the type and duration needed by persons with ALS, even if services are occurring concomitantly. Congress should grant CMS the authority to provide concomitant services at home and as an outpatient for progressive, neurodegenerative diseases such as ALS.

b. Commit to expedited (within 72 hours) responses to prior authorization requests for all therapies, durable medical equipment, assistive technologies, and services for persons with ALS.

c. Do not deny services for persons with ALS based on failure to show functional improvement, given the progressive nature of the illness.

d. Establish a call center for persons living with ALS, and possibly other rare diseases, and their caregivers to report challenges in receiving care and services.

e. Work with ALS organizations and persons living with ALS and their families to develop a "Know Your Rights" document that describes Medicare, Medicaid, and private insurance requirements and empowers individuals living with ALS to combat misinformation and improper denial of services.

Recommendation 3-2: Enable all persons with ALS to access and make full use of ALS care.

Congress should act quickly to enable all persons with ALS to access timely, specialty ALS care by doing the following:

a. Expand the status of ALS as a qualifying condition for Medicare coverage, such that persons with ALS are eligible for Medicare coverage regardless of age, employment history, or other criteria influencing Medicare or Social Security Disability Insurance eligibility.

b. Require reimbursement of multidisciplinary ALS care under a bundled payment method commensurate with the services provided.

Recommendation 3-3: Provide centralized resources for people with ALS to receive support for needs not otherwise accessible or covered by insurance. ALS nonprofit organizations and patient-serving associations should collaborate to create and maintain centralized resources to guide people with ALS and their caregivers to organizations and funding mechanisms that can provide financial support for needs not otherwise accessible to them or covered by Medicare, Medicaid, and private insurance. These might include such things as mental health services, modifications to home environments, securing equipment and assistive technologies, and transportation.

SUPPORTING CAREGIVERS

The term *caregiver* typically refers to a family member or other individual who supports someone living with ALS. These caregivers are sometimes called *informal* or *unpaid* caregivers. This report uses the term *unpaid caregiver* to encompass the individual—family member or other individual—primarily caring for and supporting the individual living with ALS. While *informal caregiver* is frequently used in the literature, the committee heard that this terminology conveys something "casual" or "not done to the highest standards" which could diminish their important work for individuals with ALS.

ALS requires a high intensity of care at home, and as a result, caregivers face their own unique challenges (Poppe et al., 2020; Williams et al., 2008) (see Box 3-1). The physical demands of caring for someone with ALS are substantial and range from assistance with activities of daily living such as bathing, using the bathroom, eating, and dressing to managing mobility aids (Young et al., 2023). Eventually, the person living with ALS will need feeding devices and breathing machines. In addition, the spouse or other family member of a person living with ALS often manages the household, including child care, cleaning, doing laundry, paying bills, making health care provider appointments, and communicating with other family members.

The challenge of caring for a person living with ALS can lead to depression, anxiety, and other impairments (de Wit et al., 2018). Caregiver burnout is a serious risk as the patient's condition deteriorates, the responsibilities of care increase, and the hours spent caring for the individual increase (Shan et al., 2021). Studies have shown that psychological distress, hours of care provided, and lower quality of life were significant predictors of higher caregiver burden (Markella Antoniadi et al., 2020; Galvin et al., 2016).

The quality of life of individuals with ALS is also highly intertwined with the quality of life of their caregivers. The well-being of caregivers, typically providing unpaid care in the patient's home, is challenged as their role as a caregiver evolves (Poppe et al., 2020; Williams et al., 2008). From the time of diagnosis to the disease's terminal phase, the caregiver assumes many roles: engaging with professional clinical care providers to develop a care plan; navigating insurance; coordinating medical

---

BOX 3-1
Perspectives from Caregivers of People Living with ALS

"From a caregiver standpoint, it's just a lot. A lot of challenges."
—*Syliva Clingman, caregiver of a person living with ALS*

"When we received the diagnosis, it was horrible. We were called by her neurologist and given the information over the phone, but no support. With that information, I was left to try to console myself, console my daughter and figure out what are the next steps, without any support from the doctor who provided us with the diagnosis or any support from anyone from the hospital, whether it would have been a social worker or someone from the ALS clinic at that point. . . . Mental health is a key factor when taking care of a loved one with a terminal illness. ALS crippled my beloved daughter and watching that day in and day out has taken a toll on me. I watched my daughter deteriorate over time and there was nothing I could do but show up every day and give her 100% of my attention in regards to her caregiving. I did not have time to sit back and grieve what was actually happening to her."
—*Vanessa Jackson, Mother/caregiver of person living/passed away from ALS*

"I have never had help that I could rely on enough to keep employed outside the home, so that has also been a big thing for me, and that will be my biggest concern after, is that I will have a large employment gap and no income or help as I adjust to creating income and establishing basically a whole new life after."
—*Ashley Lee, caregiver of a person living with ALS*

SOURCE: Presented by Sylvia Clingman, Vanessa Jackson, and Ashley Lee at "Amyotrophic Lateral Sclerosis: Accelerating Treatments and Improving Quality of Life - #2" on August 23, 2023.

---

equipment acquisition; coordinating in-home paid formal care providers; and often learning to monitor complicated, life-sustaining equipment such as ventilators. The ability of the unpaid caregiver to accomplish these tasks can be severely hampered by a lack of adequate resources and supports. Instructions from clinicians, insurers, or DME manufacturers can be rare, and even when it is available, it can be difficult to access. For example, telephone help lines and servicing for DME may not be available around the clock.

A scoping review of 37 studies examined the supportive care needs of individuals living with ALS and their caregivers and identified many deficits (Oh and Kim, 2017). The most common domain areas of unmet needs were categorized into the seven domains of the Supportive Care Needs Framework:[10] practical, informational, social, psychological, physical, emotional, and spiritual. For example, as described earlier in this chapter, individuals living with ALS who have Medicare or private insurance often face complex, demoralizing insurance processes such as prior authorization requirements for services and assistive technologies that are always medically indicated given the very nature of the progressive disease. In these situations, unmet needs in most, if not all, of these support care areas exacerbate the challenges to a person living with ALS and their caregiver's quality of life.

The hours devoted to unpaid caregiving are substantial. A 2021 ALSA survey found that 68 percent of those surveyed spent more than 30 hours per week providing care (ALS Focus, 2021). Unpaid caregivers can spend more than 100 hours per week providing care (Kennedy et al., 2022; MNDA, 2016). A large multicenter study at three European sites reported in 2021 that unpaid caregivers in each of three community-based cohorts devoted an average of 35 to 97 hours per week to their duties (Conroy et al., 2021). A 2022 study conducted through ALSA of British Columbia examining the effects of respite care found unpaid caregivers provided on average of 65.3 hours of care per week (Wu et al., 2022). Although advances in other aspects of ALS disease management, including drug therapy and digital technologies, have occurred over the past 20 years, there has been no reduction in the time people with ALS require of their family caregivers. Reports from European and Australian cohorts in 2003 and 2012, respectively, found that just over 12 hours per day was spent tending to the care recipient (Aoun et al., 2012; Kaub-Wittemer et al., 2003).

The time devoted to caregiving, combined with the lack of adequate support, contributes to the high level of distress experienced by the unpaid care provider (Oh and Kim, 2017). Documentation of high caregiver burden is noted in studies from various populations (Conroy et al., 2021; de Wit et al., 2019; Galvin et al., 2018; Larsson et al., 2022; Schischlevskij et al., 2021). The consequences for the unpaid care providers include greater risk of depression and other psychological symptoms (de Wit et al., 2019) and significant impairment of their own physical health (Schischlevskij et al., 2021).

Respite care, a service that provides family caregivers with time away from their caregiving responsibilities, can improve the emotional and physical health of a caregiver. Paying for respite care can be a challenge, as few insurance plans will pay for it. Medicare covers 95 percent of the cost of

---

[10]See Fitch, 2008.

respite care in approved facilities as part of its hospice benefit for those indi-viduals with ALS who have elected to enroll in a hospice program. Outside of the hospice benefit, Medicare does not cover respite services, but some Medi-care Advantage plans may cover respite services. Some states have a respite voucher program, and some states' Medicaid policies cover respite care.

For veterans, the U.S. Department of Veterans Affairs (VA) covers up to 30 days of respite care annually through the Program for Comprehensive Assistance to Family Caregivers. Faith-based organizations and charitable organizations may provide financial support to offset the costs of respite services, and funds may be available through the National Family Caregiver Support Program administered by local Area Agencies on Aging. Beyond paying for respite care, caregivers for individuals living with ALS also reported to the committee the added challenge of finding qualified, trust-worthy respite care providers they felt comfortable leaving the individual living with ALS in their care for an extended period. Given that caring for an individual living with ALS can require understanding and monitor-ing complex communication or respiratory devices, only individuals with proper training and experience would be qualified to provide respite care.

Models of Caregiver Support

There are numerous models for supporting caregivers, and federal policy continues to evolve to further meet their needs. For example, CMS has reaffirmed the responsibility of hospitals to engage caregivers in hospi-tal discharge processes and post-acute settings. CMS will also now provide payment when practitioners (physician or nonphysician) train caregivers to support individuals with certain diseases or illnesses in carrying out a treatment plan (CMS, 2023b).

The committee believes the following two models, if adapted for people with ALS and their caregivers, could address the challenges that those who care for family members with ALS face.

U.S. Department of Veterans Affairs Caregiver Support Program

The VA has a Caregiver Support Program (CSP) with a CSP team at every VA facility offering clinical services to caregivers of eligible and cov-ered veterans. Veterans can designate one primary family caregiver and up to two secondary family caregivers for eligibility in the program. Primary caregivers receive:

- Monthly stipend paid directly to the caregiver;
- Access to health insurance through VA if they do not already have health insurance;

- Mental health counseling;
- Certain beneficiary travel benefits when traveling with the veteran to appointments; and
- At least 30 days of respite care per year, for the veteran.

Secondary caregivers do not receive a monthly stipend but are eligible for certain travel benefits when traveling with the veteran to appointments and mental health counseling.

Guiding an Improved Dementia Experience (GUIDE) Model

In response to the Biden administration's April 2023 Increasing Access to High-Quality Care and Supporting Caregivers Executive Order, CMS initiated a test of a new voluntary, nationwide model program that supports people living with dementia and their unpaid caregivers.[11] People living with dementia receive fragmented care and often have multiple chronic conditions, leading to high rates of hospitalization and emergency department visits. In addition, people with dementia often have round-the-clock care needs and behavioral and psychological symptoms. Caregivers for people living with dementia report high levels of stress and depression, which negatively affect their overall health and increase their risk for serious illness, hospitalization, and mortality.

The GUIDE model will test an alternative payment for participants, such as dementia care programs comprising an interdisciplinary team, that provides ongoing, longitudinal care and support to people living with dementia. The model aims to address the key drivers of poor-quality dementia care in five ways (CMS, 2023c):

1. Define a standardized approach to dementia care delivery for model participants. This includes staffing considerations, services for beneficiaries and their unpaid caregivers, and quality standards.
2. Provide an alternative payment methodology to model participants. CMS will provide a monthly per-beneficiary payment to support a team-based collaborative approach.
3. Address unpaid caregiver needs. The model will aim to address the burden experienced by unpaid caregivers by requiring model participants to provide caregiver training and support services, including 24/7 access to a support line and connections to community-based providers.
4. Offer respite services. CMS will pay model participants for respite services provided to a beneficiary in their home, at an adult day

---

[11]At the time of this report's writing, the GUIDE model had been announced and applications were under review. The model is scheduled to launch on July 1, 2024, and run for 8 years.

center, or at a facility that can provide 24-hour care for the purpose of giving the unpaid caregiver temporary breaks from their caregiving responsibilities.
5. Screen for health-related social needs. Model participants will be required to screen beneficiaries for psychosocial needs and health-related social needs and help navigate them to local community-based organizations to address these needs.

Since the GUIDE model was developed for people with dementia and their caregivers, not all of the above will apply to people with ALS or their caregivers. For example, caregivers for people with ALS might require training from clinicians, home health agencies, DME manufacturers, and community organizations. These support needs might evolve as the care needs of the person with ALS also progress; they might, for instance, require training for a ventilator, a power wheelchair, or a home or vehicle modification at different times. Because of these complex and developing needs, CMS might extend stipends to pay for caregiver training.

Palliative Care to Improve Quality of Life for Persons with ALS and Caregivers

Palliative care is a field of medicine focused on improving quality of life for patients with serious life-limiting illnesses. Neuropalliative care is a specialty of palliative care for patients with neurological disorders and plays a critical role in improving quality of life for individuals living with ALS and their care partners (Brizzi et al., 2019; Phillips et al., 2020). An American Academy of Neurology Ethics and Humanities Committee position statement highlighted the ethical responsibilities of neurologists to their patients, stating,

> It is imperative that neurologists understand and learn to apply the principles of palliative care as . . . many patients with neurologic disease die after long illnesses during which the neurologist acts as the principal or consulting physician. (Taylor et al., 2022)

ALSA has also highlighted the importance of providing palliative care to people living with ALS attending an ALS multidisciplinary clinic. Some of the most troublesome ALS symptoms palliative care manages include pain, cramps, spasticity, breathing difficulties, excessive saliva flow, episodes of sudden uncontrollable and inappropriate laughing or crying, and depression. Integrating a palliative care specialist into a multidisciplinary care system can facilitate care delivery by reducing the travel burden to patients and caregivers.

Financial, time, and resource constraints often hamper comprehensive care that includes palliative care (Kluger et al., 2023). Integrating neuropalliative care within the multidisciplinary care model—during regular clinical visits through templates and checklists, for example (Kluger et al., 2023)—will require better resource allocation and additional workforce. Other barriers to palliative care include lack of awareness among policy makers, health professionals, and patients about palliative care and its benefits. There also are misconceptions that palliative care is only for patients with cancer or those at the end of life, and is sometimes confused with hospice. Finally, there is no downside to receiving palliative care.

Hospice and Palliative Care

Patients become eligible for hospice care when they are expected to live fewer than 6 months. Most U.S. hospice care is provided by Medicare's hospice program. Private insurance plans may also provide hospice care for patients who do not qualify for Medicare hospice. Most multidisciplinary hospice care occurs at the patient's residence and occasionally in a long-term care facility. Persons with ALS may have hospice enrollment extended when there is documented evidence of continued progress of terminal disease. Individuals receiving palliative care may be transitioned to Medicare hospice care when the prognosis is 6 months or less.

Elevating and Responding to the Needs of ALS Caregivers

Caregivers for persons with ALS need significant levels of support from a variety of providers that can span diverse and different venues. VA provides substantial supports to caregivers for veterans with ALS and the committee believes similar supports and financial resources should be available to all caregivers for persons with ALS. To meet these needs, the committee offers the following recommendation.

Recommendation 3-4: Address the needs of unpaid caregivers.

Congress, the Centers for Medicare & Medicaid Services (CMS), private insurers, and ALS organizations should address the needs of unpaid caregivers, including respite care, reimbursement for caregiving, and mental and other health support services, including the following:
> **a.** **National and local ALS nonprofits should collaborate to develop a priority list of caregiver needs to inform collective advocacy efforts of national ALS nonprofits. This could be accompanied by a guide for ALS caregivers on what to expect through the course of disease and identify resources, which would be used by all national nonprofits and updated collaboratively.**

b. Congress should provide financial support for caregivers by amending the tax code to provide a tax credit that could be used by caregivers for individuals living with ALS, as well as all progressive neurodegenerative diseases to alleviate the financial burden of providing unpaid care. Congress should also provide other types of financial relief for caregivers, including allowing them to apply health savings account or flexible spending account funds to caring for a parent or parent-in-law.

c. CMS should ensure legally covered services for home health aides are accessible.

d. CMS should expand tests of payment and service delivery models, such as the Guiding an Improved Dementia Experience model for people with dementia and their caregivers, to include ALS, or create new programs specifically designed to support persons with ALS and their unpaid caregivers. These tests should include:

- Stipends paid directly to caregivers on an at least a monthly basis,
- Reimbursing persons with ALS and their caregivers for accessing mental health counseling and psychotherapy via video telehealth (across state lines), and
- Access to high-quality respite care services.

RESPIRATORY MANAGEMENT OF ALS

Most deaths from ALS result from respiratory failure, making early recognition of respiratory impairment and longitudinal management of chronic respiratory failure critical to improve both quality and quantity of life for individuals living with ALS (Khan et al., 2023; Miller et al., 2009). ALS leads to weakness of the diaphragm and respiratory muscles resulting in progressive and unrelenting shortness of breath exacerbated by impaired cough mechanisms. Increased risk of aspiration of secretions and pneumonia can lead to increased hospitalizations.

In the United States, clinicians use pulmonary function tests (PFTs) to detect and quantify impaired lung physiology and diaphragm weakness. PFTs allow clinicians to identify those people living with ALS who will benefit most from respiratory support in the form of noninvasive mechanical ventilation (NIV) or home mechanical ventilation (HMV).[12,13] NIV uses

---

[12]Many other developed countries rely on a simple symptom-based approach rather than PFTs, allowing for earlier initiation of NIV or HMV.

[13]Some individuals living with ALS choose to have a tracheostomy to receive home ventilation later in disease progression.

a respiratory device that assists and augments the mechanics of breathing to reduce dyspnea, the sensation of running out of air and not being able to breathe fast or deeply enough. Respiratory support using NIV prolongs survival and improves or maintains quality of life (Bourke et al., 2006; Radunovic et al., 2017). Failing to provide NIV for individuals with ALS is no longer justifiable (Ackrivo, 2023; Radunovic et al., 2017; Rimmer et al., 2019). Research is needed, however, to determine the optimal timing and criteria for initiating NIV, although randomized controlled trials are difficult given it is unethical to withhold NIV from a control group (Radunovic et al., 2017; Rimmer et al., 2019).

Assistive ventilation to support diaphragm and respiratory muscle weakness, cough assist devices to clear airway and respiratory secretions, longitudinal monitoring of PFTs,[14] and attentive adjustment of NIV or HMV to match the progressive decline of respiratory strength are the pillars of optimal respiratory management for individuals with ALS (Ackrivo, 2023; Hansen-Flaschen and Ackrivo, 2023). However, managing comprehensive respiratory care is time and labor intensive, requiring attentive home care to optimize multiple medical equipment devices, coordination with pulmonologists with expertise in management of complex mechanical ventilators, and working with DME companies to maintain high-quality, longitudinal respiratory care (Ackrivo, 2023; Hansen-Flaschen and Ackrivo, 2023). In addition, several other factors complicate providing assistive ventilation for people living with ALS, including:

- Current Medicare policy requires an individual to have a forced vital capacity of less than 50 percent before initiating NIV or HMV therapy. A forced vital capacity of less than 50 percent means someone has significant respiratory impairment and severe shortness of breath. This leads to many people living with ALS not qualifying for NIV until they are severely symptomatic with extremes of shortness of breath. Other international guidelines have expanded criteria for NIV, focusing on an earlier symptom-based management approach that allows people living with ALS to proactively benefit from NIV or HMV support earlier in their disease (Wolfe et al., 2021).
- Commercial insurance companies make it difficult, or impossible, for individuals living with ALS to receive the respiratory devices they need. For example, it has been reported that one United Healthcare plan offered under Medicare Advantage denied 86 percent of prior authorization requests for NIV devices prescribed by physicians for individuals living with ALS (Balas, 2024).

---

[14]Clinical practice guidelines suggest closely monitoring PFTs at a minimum of 6-month intervals (Khan et al., 2023).

- Challenges exist because of the limited number of health care providers trained in chronic respiratory failure expertise.
- A lack of home support to assist caregivers with the burden of managing all that goes into providing respiratory care at home, such as cough assist, suctioning secretions, and attending to mechanical ventilators and tracheostomy.
- There is a paucity of research trials relevant to respiratory care for individuals living with ALS. With marked advancements in medical technology, home-based respiratory care therapy creates the opportunity to study and understand models of care that allow people living with ALS to maintain their quality of life at home.

Opportunities to Improve Respiratory Care for Individuals Living with ALS

There are many opportunities to optimize respiratory care for people living with respiratory impairment from ALS. VA has demonstrated exemplary comprehensive care for persons with ALS and care partners, particularly in providing comprehensive respiratory care support. Thanks to technological advancements, home ventilation and home physiology monitoring of ventilation and oxygenation now rivals physiologic monitoring performed in intensive care units, enabling persons with ALS to benefit from advances in respiratory management in the comfort of their home. Despite evidence that proactive, respiratory management prolongs survival and improves quality of life, there are several barriers to delivering optimal clinical respiratory care for persons with ALS, including:

- Inconsistencies and uncertainties exist around policies for HMV and backup ventilators to guarantee 24 hours of ventilatory support in Medicare Advantage and commercial insurance plans.
- Insurance plans can limit access to life-saving and life-supporting NIV or HMV devices for persons with ALS. The lengthy and complex prior authorization adjudication process for services, such as receiving physical therapy outside of the multidisciplinary clinic, and equipment, including power wheelchairs and ventilation at home, unnecessarily increases stress, anxiety, and the overall burden of the disease for persons with ALS. ALS multidisciplinary care teams spend many unreimbursed, unaccounted hours on prior authorization requests for equipment needed to care for a person with ALS.
- There is an insufficient number of providers trained in chronic respiratory failure. Opportunities exist to create a new subspecialty in pulmonary medicine devoted to chronic respiratory failure to meet the evolving needs of persons living with ALS (Cao et al., 2024).

- Sufficient supports for caregivers to persons with ALS are lacking. Caregivers face the challenge of managing everything required for respiratory care at home, such as cough assist, suctioning secretions, and attending to mechanical ventilators and tracheostomy.

The committee believes that a diagnosis of ALS and the very nature of the disease is sufficient justification for an individual to access respiratory devices. There is strong scientific evidence to support the earlier initiation of respiratory intervention for individuals living with ALS than is currently allowed under Medicare policy (i.e., the CMS requirement of a forced vital capacity of less than 50 percent). Individuals living with ALS need earlier access to respiratory devices as well as high-quality respiratory care from qualified providers through a multidisciplinary ALS clinic and at home. A unique opportunity exists to quickly update CMS and other insurer policies to align with the scientific evidence and develop reimbursement models for respiratory therapy to be provided in the home.

The American Academy of Neurology recommends involving respiratory therapists in multidisciplinary ALS care to optimize home respiratory management (Miller et al., 2009). Respiratory therapists have the expertise to educate patients and caregivers regarding optimal management of assisted ventilation and cough assistance strategies to allow patients to remain at home, thereby improving their quality of life and satisfaction and reducing unnecessary hospitalizations (Ackrivo, 2023; Hansen-Flaschen and Ackrivo, 2023; Khan et al., 2023). Home respiratory care is not reimbursed, but if reimbursement were expanded to include home patient care, respiratory therapists could substantially improve the quality of home respiratory care management. In addition, there is a marked lack of pulmonary physicians trained in the management of chronic respiratory failure due to neuromuscular conditions and strategies to increase this area are imperative to optimize longitudinal respiratory care (Cao et al., 2024).

However, as discussed earlier, a common barrier to respiratory care is delayed access to HMV. Current Medicare and insurance guidelines preclude acquisition of home ventilation until a person experiences 50 percent reduction in lung function, which leaves persons with ALS distressed with profound shortness of breath (Wolfe et al., 2021). Therefore, CMS should update payment policies to allow for access to home ventilation, consistent with guidance from pulmonary, respiratory therapy, and sleep medicine professional groups and accepted international standards (Wolfe et al., 2021).

Recommendation 3-5: Enable access to respiratory devices and services for people with ALS.

The Centers for Medicare & Medicaid Services (CMS) and private insurers should immediately align coverage of respiratory devices and services for persons with ALS with the current standard of care. CMS and private insurers should also develop reimbursement models that allow respiratory professionals to provide high-quality, longitudinal respiratory care in the home of a person with ALS.

REFERENCES

Ackrivo, J. 2023. Pulmonary care for ALS: Progress, gaps, and paths forward. *Muscle Nerve* 67(5):341–353.

ALS Focus. 2021. ALS *Focus results from the caregiver needs survey.* Arlington, VA: ALS Association.

ALSA (ALS Association). 2021. *ALS Focus results from the mobility survey.* Arlington, VA: ALS Association.

ALSA. 2023a. Making the challenging a little less so—your ALS care team and health insurance. In *ALSA Blog.* https://www.als.org/blog/making-challenging-little-less-so-your-als-care-team-and-health-insurance (accessed April 3, 2024).

ALSA. 2023b. *ALS focus results: Insurance and payment for ALS care.* Arlington, VA: ALS Association.

ALSA. 2024. Navigating insurance denials: A major hurdle for people living with ALS. In *ALSA Blog.* https://www.als.org/blog/navigating-insurance-denials-major-hurdle-people-living-als (accessed April 18, 2024).

AMA (American Medical Association). 2022. *Measuring progress in improving prior authorization: 2022 update.* https://www.ama-assn.org/system/files/prior-authorization-reform-progress-update.pdf (accessed March 6, 2024).

Aoun, S. M., S. L. Connors, L. Priddis, L. J. Breen, and S. Colyer. 2012. Motor neurone disease family carers' experiences of caring, palliative care and bereavement: An exploratory qualitative study. *Palliative Med* 26(6):842–850.

Balas, C. 2024. *Why Medicare Advantage plans continue to deny life-saving ventilators to ALS patients.* https://www.ibtimes.com/why-medicare-advantage-plans-continues-deny-life-saving-ventilators-als-patients-3721592 (accessed March 6, 2024).

Bourke, S. C., M. Tomlinson, T. L. Williams, R. E. Bullock, P. J. Shaw, and G. J. Gibson. 2006. Effects of non-invasive ventilation on survival and quality of life in patients with amyotrophic lateral sclerosis: A randomised controlled trial. *Lancet Neurol* 5(2):140–147.

Brizzi, K., S. Paganoni, A. Zehm, F. De Marchi, and J. D. Berry. 2019. Integration of a palliative care specialist in an amyotrophic lateral sclerosis clinic: Observations from one center. *Muscle Nerve* 60(2):137–140.

Cao, M., S. L. Katz, and J. Hansen-Flaschen. 2024. Roadmap for advancing a new subspecialty in pulmonary medicine devoted to chronic respiratory failure. *Ann Am Thorac Soc* 21(5):692–695.

Center for Medicare Advocacy. 2013. *Self-help packet for home health care appeals including "improvement standard" denials.* https://medicareadvocacy.org/self-help-packet-for-expedited-home-health-care-appeals-including-improvement-standard-denials (accessed March 6, 2024).

Center for Medicare Advocacy. 2016. *Medicare: Time to renew not retreat.* Willimantic, CT: Center for Medicare Advocacy.

Center for Medicare Advocacy. 2018. *Medicare home health coverage in light of* Jimmo v. Sebelius: *You do not have to improve to qualify for Medicare coverage.* Willimantic, CT: Center for Medicare Advocacy.

Certner, D. 2023. Re: CMS–1780–P. Medicare program. https://www.aarp.org/content/dam/aarp/ politics/advocacy/2023/08/home-health-payment-comments.pdf (accessed August 28, 2023).

CMS (Centers for Medicare & Medicaid Services). 2023a. *Seat elevation systems as an accessory to power wheelchairs (group 3)*. https://www.cms.gov/medicare-coverage-database/view/ ncacal-decision-memo.aspx?proposed=N&ncaid=309 (accessed May 22, 2024).

CMS. 2023b. *Calendar year (CY) 2024 Medicare physician fee schedule final rule*. https:// www.cms.gov/newsroom/fact-sheets/calendar-year-cy-2024-medicare-physician-fee- schedule-final-rule (accessed May 21, 2024).

CMS. 2023c. *Guiding an Improved Dementia Experience (GUIDE) model*. https://www.cms.gov/ priorities/innovation/innovation-models/guide (accessed March 6, 2024).

Conroy, É., P. Kennedy, M. Heverin, I. Leroi, E. Mayberry, A. Beelen, T. Stavroulakis, L. H. van den Berg, C. J. McDermott, O. Hardiman, and M. Galvin. 2021. Informal caregivers in amyotrophic lateral sclerosis: A multi-centre, exploratory study of burden and difficulties. *Brain Sci* 11(8).

Cubanski, J. N., T. Neuman, and M. Freed. 2023. *Explaining the prescription drug provisions in the Inflation Reduction Act*. https://www.kff.org/medicare/issue-brief/explaining-the- prescription-drug-provisions-in-the-inflation-reduction-act (accessed March 10, 2024).

de Wit, J., L. A. Bakker, A. C. van Groenestijn, L. H. van den Berg, C. D. Schroder, J. M. A. Visser-Meily, and A. Beelen. 2018. Caregiver burden in amyotrophic lateral sclerosis: A systematic review. *Palliative Med* 32(1):231–245.

de Wit, J., L. A. Bakker, A. C. van Groenestijn, J. F. Baardman, L. H. van den Berg, J. M. A. Visser-Meily, and C. D. Schröder. 2019. Psychological distress and coping styles of care- givers of patients with amyotrophic lateral sclerosis: A longitudinal study. *Amyotroph Lateral Scler Frontotemporal Degener* 20(3–4):235–241.

Fitch, M. I. 2008. Supportive care framework. *Can Oncol Nurs J* 18(1):6–24.

Friedman, A., J. Howard, E. K. Shaw, D. J. Cohen, L. Shahidi, and J. M. Ferrante. 2016. Fa- cilitators and barriers to care coordination in patient-centered medical homes (PCMHs) from coordinators' perspectives. *J Am Board Fam Med* 29(1):90–101.

Galvin, C., W. Yang, and A. Saadi. 2023. Evaluation of crowdsourced fundraising to cover health care costs for neurological conditions in the US. *JAMA Neurol* 80(9):1000–1002.

Galvin, M., B. Corr, C. Madden, I. Mays, R. McQuillan, V. Timonen, A. Staines, and O. Hardiman. 2016. Caregiving in ALS—a mixed methods approach to the study of burden. *BMC Palliative Care* 15(1):81.

Galvin, M., S. Carney, B. Corr, I. Mays, N. Pender, and O. Hardiman. 2018. Needs of informal caregivers across the caregiving course in amyotrophic lateral sclerosis: A qualitative analysis. *BMJ Open* 8(1):e018721.

Gelinas, L., E. A. Largent, I. G. Cohen, S. Kornetsky, B. E. Bierer, and H. Fernandez Lynch. 2018. A framework for ethical payment to research participants. *N Engl J Med* 378(8):766–771.

Gladman, M., and L. Zinman. 2015. The economic impact of amyotrophic lateral sclerosis: A systematic review. *Expert Rev Pharmacoecon Outcomes Res* 15(3):439–450.

Hansen-Flaschen, J., and J. Ackrivo. 2023. Practical guide to management of long-term non- invasive ventilation for adults with chronic neuromuscular disease. *Respiratory Care* 68(8):1123–1157.

Kaub-Wittemer, D., N. Steinbüchel, M. Wasner, G. Laier-Groeneveld, and G. D. Borasio. 2003. Quality of life and psychosocial issues in ventilated patients with amyotrophic lateral sclerosis and their caregivers. *J Pain Sympt Manag* 26(4):890–896.

Kennedy, P., É. Conroy, M. Heverin, I. Leroi, A. Beelen, L. van den Berg, O. Hardiman, and M. Galvin. 2022. Burden and benefit—A mixed methods study of informal amyotrophic lateral sclerosis caregivers in Ireland and the Netherlands. *Int J Geriatr Psychiatry* 37(5).

Khan, A., L. Frazer-Green, R. Amin, L. Wolfe, G. Faulkner, K. Casey, G. Sharma, B. Selim, D. Zielinski, L. S. Aboussouan, D. McKim, and P. Gay. 2023. Respiratory management of patients with neuromuscular weakness: An American College of Chest Physicians clinical practice guideline and expert panel report. *Chest* 164(2):394–413.

King, R. S. 2024. Caregivers helped us be a family. Everyone should have that option. *New York Times*, January 8, 2024.

Kluger, B. M., P. Hudson, L. C. Hanson, R. Bužgovà, C. J. Creutzfeldt, R. Gursahani, M. Sumrall, C. White, D. J. Oliver, S. Z. Pantilat, and J. Miyasaki. 2023. Palliative care to support the needs of adults with neurological disease. *Lancet Neurol* 22(7):619–631.

Korbey, M. 2023. *People with ALS can get Social Security disability benefits sooner.* https://blog.ssa.gov/people-with-als-can-get-social-security-disability-benefits-sooner (accessed March 6, 2024).

Larsson, B. J., A. Ozanne, K. Nordin, and I. Nygren. 2022. Quality of life among relatives of patients with amyotrophic lateral sclerosis: A prospective and longitudinal study. *Palliative Supportive Care* 20(2):203–211.

Markella Antoniadi, A., M. Galvin, M. Heverin, O. Hardiman, and C. Mooney. 2020. Prediction of caregiver burden in amyotrophic lateral sclerosis: A machine learning approach using random forests applied to a cohort study. *BMJ Open* 10(2):e033109.

Miller, R. G., C. E. Jackson, E. J. Kasarskis, J. D. England, D. Forshew, W. Johnston, S. Kalra, J. S. Katz, H. Mitsumoto, J. Rosenfeld, C. Shoesmith, M. J. Strong, and S. C. Woolley. 2009. Practice parameter update: The care of the patient with amyotrophic lateral sclerosis: Multidisciplinary care, symptom management, and cognitive/behavioral impairment (an evidence-based review). Report of the Quality Standards Subcommittee of the American Academy of Neurology. *Neurology* 73(15):1227–1233.

MNDA (Motor Neurone Disease Association). 2016. *Caring for carers of people with MND: How government can help.* Northampton, UK: Motor Neurone Disease Association.

Möckli, N., M. Simon, C. Meyer-Massetti, S. Pihet, R. Fischer, M. Wächter, C. Serdaly, and F. Zúñiga. 2021. Factors associated with homecare coordination and quality of care: A research protocol for a national multi-center cross-sectional study. *BMC Health Serv Res* 21(1):306.

Obermann, M., and M. Lyon. 2015. Financial cost of amyotrophic lateral sclerosis: A case study. *Amyotroph Lateral Scler Frontotemp Degener* 16(1–2):54–57.

Oh, J., and J. A. Kim. 2017. Supportive care needs of patients with amyotrophic lateral sclerosis/motor neuron disease and their caregivers: A scoping review. *J Clin Nurs* 26(23–24):4129–4152.

Phillips, J. N., J. Besbris, L. A. Foster, N. M. Kramer, S. Maiser, and A. K. Mehta. 2020. Models of outpatient neuropalliative care for patients with amyotrophic lateral sclerosis. *Neurol* 95(17):782–788.

Poppe, C., I. Kone, L. M. Iseli, K. Schweikert, B. S. Elger, and T. Wangmo. 2020. Differentiating needs of informal caregivers of individuals with ALS across the caregiving course: A systematic review. *Amyotroph Lateral Scler Frontotemp Degener* 21(7–8):519–541.

Radunovic, A., D. Annane, M. K. Rafiq, R. Brassington, and N. Mustfa. 2017. Mechanical ventilation for amyotrophic lateral sclerosis/motor neuron disease. *Cochrane Database System Rev* 10:CD004427.

Rimmer, K. P., M. Kaminska, M. Nonoyama, E. Giannouli, F. Maltais, D. L. Morrison, C. O'Connell, B. J. Petrof, and D. A. McKim. 2019. Home mechanical ventilation for patients with amyotrophic lateral sclerosis: A Canadian Thoracic Society clinical practice guideline. *Can J Respir, Crit Care, Sleep Med* 3(1):9–27.

Schischlevskij, P., I. Cordts, R. Günther, B. Stolte, D. Zeller, C. Schröter, U. Weyen, M. Regensburger, J. Wolf, I. Schneider, A. Hermann, M. Metelmann, Z. Kohl, R. A. Linker, J. C. Koch, C. Stendel, L. H. Müschen, A. Osmanovic, C. Binz, T. Klopstock, J. Dorst, A. C. Ludolph, M. Boentert, T. Hagenacker, M. Deschauer, P. Lingor, S. Petri, and O. Schreiber-Katz. 2021. Informal caregiving in amyotrophic lateral sclerosis (ALS): A high caregiver burden and drastic consequences on caregivers' lives. *Brain Sci* 11(6).

Shan, T., L. Li, X. Hongxia, C. Shuyan, L. Chao, H. Kunjing, and W. Binquan. 2021. Caregiver burden and associated factors among primary caregivers of patients with ALS in home care: A cross-sectional survey study. *BMJ Open* 11(9):e050185.

Tang, S., Li, L., Xue, H., Cao, S., Li, C., Han, K., Wang, B.. 2021. Caregiver burden and associated factors among primary caregivers of patients with ALS in home care: A cross-sectional survey study. *BMJ Open* 11(9):e050185.

Taylor, L. P., J. M. Besbris, W. D. Graf, M. A. Rubin, S. Cruz-Flores, and L. G. Epstein. 2022. Clinical guidance in neuropalliative care. *Neurology* 98(10):409–416.

Williams, M. T., J. P. Donnelly, T. Holmlund, and M. Battaglia. 2008. ALS: Family caregiver needs and quality of life. *Amyotroph Lateral Scler* 9(5):279–286.

Wolfe, L. F., J. O. Benditt, L. Aboussouan, D. R. Hess, and J. M. Coleman, 3rd. 2021. Optimal NIV Medicare access promotion: Patients with thoracic restrictive disorders: A technical expert panel report from the American College of Chest Physicians, the American Association for Respiratory Care, the American Academy of Sleep Medicine, and the American Thoracic Society. *Chest* 160(5):e399–e408.

Wu, J. M., M. T. Tam, K. Buch, F. Khairati, L. Wilson, E. Bannerman, A. Guerrero, A. Eisen, W. Toyer, T. Stevenson, and J. M. Robillard. 2022. The impact of respite care from the perspectives and experiences of people with amyotrophic lateral sclerosis and their care partners: A qualitative study. *BMC Palliative Care* 21(1):26.

Young, H. M., T. R. Kilaberia, R. Whitney, B. M. Link, J. F. Bell, O. Tonkikh, J. Famula, and B. Oskarsson. 2023. Needs of persons living with ALS at home and their family caregivers: A scoping review. *Muscle Nerve* 68(3):240–249.

4

Creating a Sustainable and Accessible ALS Clinical Care and Research System

ABSTRACT

This chapter discusses the importance of establishing an integrated, nationwide system of care and research for individuals living with amyotrophic lateral sclerosis (ALS) as well as at-risk genetic carriers. The two goals for this system will be (1) to ensure all individuals with ALS and at-risk genetic carriers, regardless of where they live and the resources at their disposal, have equal access to high-quality, evidence-based care, and (2) for such care to be integrated with research, including health services, care delivery research, and clinical research to develop biomarkers and new therapeutics. This is important, as the number of individuals diagnosed and living with ALS in the United States continues to rise. The care and research system should build on existing facilities and ultimately constitute an integrated network linking comprehensive, regional, and community or local ALS centers. Each network level should have defined clinical care services and research capabilities and be held accountable for reducing access delays in their area, reaching underserved populations, and ensuring continuity of care throughout an individual's ALS disease course. Creating this network will require urgently expanding the number of clinics providing multidisciplinary care, growing and supporting the ALS multidisciplinary workforce, increasing capacity for early referrals and consultations for timely ALS diagnosis and access to personalized, standard-of-care therapies, and establishing new payment models to support the system of ALS clinics.

The committee believes that every individual living with ALS deserves early and continuous access to multidisciplinary,[1] state-of-the-art care to help them lead longer lives, remain functionally independent, and optimize overall quality of life. Multidisciplinary clinics provide coordinated, team-based management across multiple medical and allied health specialties and serve as a one-stop shop for complex multisystem diseases, such as ALS. Today, there are only around 200 multidisciplinary ALS clinics in the United States that provide high-quality care. That is too few to serve all individuals with ALS. The clinics are also insufficiently connected to coordinate the availability of specialized ALS expertise and research efforts to every person with ALS. There is also no definitive count of the number of people living with ALS today who receive evidence-based standard of care at a multidisciplinary clinic but one estimate from the ALS Association (ALSA) suggests that it is at best about half of the population.[2]

Multidisciplinary care visits require multiple hours and involve several health professionals, but this type of care is reimbursed at the same rate as a single specialist's 30- to 60-minute office visit (Paganoni et al., 2017). This places a financial strain on ALS multidisciplinary clinics, hindering their ability to hire, retain, and expand the clinic staff to meet the needs of people living with ALS and their families. Today, larger ALS clinics rely heavily on philanthropy and institutional resources, which is unsustainable, exacerbates the significant variations in resources that exist across U.S. ALS clinics, and limits access to state-of-the-art care.

People living with ALS also need easy access to participation in cutting-edge clinical research trials without prohibitive cost or travel burdens. Over the past 5 years, discoveries about ALS genetics, disease targets, and disease pathways have increased clinical trial activity and biomarker and therapeutic development. However, the ALS clinical research system is disjointed, underresourced, and not sufficiently connected to the ALS clinical care team. Furthermore, there are substantial geographic, racial and ethnic, and socioeconomic disparities in access to, and participation in, clinical

---

[1] As stated in Chapter 2, the committee notes that *interdisciplinary*, rather than *multidisciplinary*, is the more accurate term because interdisciplinary denotes that the various disciplines are coordinated toward a common and coherent approach, while multidisciplinary refers to the addition of the competencies of multiple professionals who stay within the boundaries of their fields (Choi and Pak, 2006). The Veterans Health Administration refers to the ALS interdisciplinary team in its directive on providing ALS care to veterans. The committee has chosen to use *multidisciplinary* in the report because it is the more widely used term.

[2] In an October 18, 2023, letter to the committee from the ALS Association, it is stated: "Although multidisciplinary ALS care can add nine months of life, it is woefully underfunded and often difficult to deliver. Only about half the people served at ALS Certified Treatment Centers of Excellence receive this well-established, evidence-based standard of care."

trials, expanded access programs, and clinical research overall. In addition to serving more individuals with ALS, expanding access to clinical research will be critical for accelerating therapeutic discoveries for this disease and informing timely, evidence-based health policy changes.

In this chapter, the committee lays out the current obstacles to accessing high-quality ALS care and proposes a reenvisioned, newly coordinated system of care and research accessible to every individual with ALS. The committee recommends establishing a system of care built on a hub-and-spoke model that integrates clinical research as a key pillar of care across ALS clinics, similar to the system developed for cancer care. This nationwide system of care and research will leverage existing clinical and research expertise and infrastructure, along with the latest technological resources, to provide all individuals living with ALS, regardless of geography and resources, access to high-quality, standardized, evidence-based multidisciplinary care. This integrated system of care and research will also enable all individuals living with ALS, if interested, to participate in clinical research aimed at making ALS a livable disease within the next decade. A more complete discussion on accelerating ALS therapeutic development can be found in Chapter 5; however, this chapter explains how an expanded and integrated multidisciplinary care network could also serve as the foundation for building a robust infrastructure for the natural history studies and clinical trials needed to advance therapeutic development.

The chapter also recommends innovative strategies for addressing four major challenges to expanding access to ALS care. Meeting these challenges is necessary for advancing research for ALS as well as other neurodegenerative diseases. The four challenges are:

1. Achieving equity across racial, ethnic, and geographically diverse groups by reaching more people, particularly underserved populations, and helping them gain access to early and continuous care at an ALS multidisciplinary clinic;
2. Workforce training and education to expand the ALS workforce and enhance professional education and awareness of ALS among health professionals;
3. Financing multidisciplinary care and research by implementing adequate payment and reimbursement models for multidisciplinary care and research and studying multidisciplinary care outcomes in terms of their value to people with ALS, families, clinicians, and insurers; and
4. Connecting the U.S. Department of Veterans Affairs (VA) health care system and veterans living with ALS to the broader care and research system.

ALS MULTIDISCIPLINARY CARE

A multidisciplinary clinic serves as a single site for people living with ALS, confirming diagnoses; initiating and monitoring therapies, medications, and assistive technology devices; and managing multisystem symptoms. A multidisciplinary clinic also provides specialized health and supportive services to track disease progression, improve quality of life, and prolong functional independence. These services include occupational, physical, speech and language, and respiratory therapy; nutritional support; mental and behavioral health services; and durable medical equipment (DME). A multidisciplinary clinic also provides neuropalliative care services for individualized advanced care planning based on ALS disease progression.

Numerous studies have demonstrated that multidisciplinary care decreases 1-year mortality by as much as 30 percent, reduces hospitalizations and cost of care, improves quality-of-life outcomes, and increases patient satisfaction (Boylan et al., 2015; Chiò et al., 2006; Cordesse et al., 2015; Corr et al., 1998; de Almeida et al., 2021; Driskell et al., 2019; Galvin et al., 2017; Hogden and Crook, 2017; Traynor et al., 2003). As a result, there is consensus in the field that multidisciplinary care should be the standard of care for all individuals living with ALS (Andersen et al., 2005; Hogden and Crook, 2017; Miller et al., 2009).

Variation in Access to ALS Centers

In contrast to the evidence supporting the usefulness and effectiveness of multidisciplinary care, evidence regarding the availability and use of multidisciplinary care in ALS is limited. ALSA estimates that approximately 12,000 people living with ALS receive care at a multidisciplinary clinic every year, representing about 40 percent of the overall U.S. ALS patient population, as estimated by the Centers for Disease Control and Prevention (CDC) (ALSA, 2023; Mehta et al., 2023). This 40 percent is a rough estimate that does not consider whether the care received was at a single visit or continuous, nor does it include people with ALS who receive care at a Muscular Dystrophy Association (MDA) specialty center or a VA clinic, both of which also provide multidisciplinary care for people with ALS. For comparison, the Cystic Fibrosis Foundation Patient Registry (see Chapter 5) estimates that 77 to 84 percent of people with cystic fibrosis in the United States attend a Cystic Fibrosis Foundation–certified clinic (Cromwell et al., 2023; Knapp et al., 2016).

ALSA lists 226 multidisciplinary clinics in the United States, certifying 89 of these as ALS Treatment Centers of Excellence and 18 as Recognized Treatment Centers.[3] Both ALS Treatment Centers of Excellence and Rec-

---

[3]The complete list of multidisciplinary ALS clinics is available at https://www.als.org/support/certified-centers-clinics.

BOX 4-1
ALSA Certification Process for
Treatment Centers of Excellence

ALSA designates multidisciplinary care clinics that diagnose and treat persons living with ALS as Certified Treatment Centers of Excellence if they:

1. Meet certain clinical care and treatment standards, based on the American Academy of Neurology's Practice Parameters for ALS (Miller et al., 2009);
2. Participate in ALS research and/or enable people living with ALS to participate in clinical trials; and
3. Pass a comprehensive clinical and administrative review performed by ALSA.

ognized Treatment Centers must meet certain standards regarding the care they provide (see Box 4-1). However, Recognized Treatment Centers may not offer opportunities to participate in ALS research. The other 119 are categorized as affiliated clinics, which deliver models of care other than those officially part of the ALSA Certified Center Program. These include both group and solo private practices. Alaska, Delaware, and Wyoming currently have no ALSA-affiliated treatment centers.

MDA also provides care to individuals living with ALS and their families because they usually have a care team with the skills needed to treat ALS as well as other neuromuscular diseases. MDA supports a care center network of more than 150 clinics nationwide. Some of these specifically serve people with ALS, whereas others are multidisciplinary neuromuscular clinics that care for individuals with ALS as well as other neuromuscular conditions. As of 2023, the VA system has nine ALSA certified Centers of Excellence (with three pending applications), two recognized treatment centers (with two pending applications), and 54 ALS multidisciplinary clinics.

While the literature is sparse, evidence suggests that many people living with ALS do not have access to multidisciplinary care. Specialty ALS clinics delivering multidisciplinary care are not uniformly distributed across the United States (see Figure 4-1), and travel distance to a multidisciplinary clinic is a commonly reported barrier for many people living with ALS (Schellenberg and Hansen, 2018; Stephens et al., 2015). A spatial analysis of 2013 data from the National ALS Registry found that 44.9 percent of people living with ALS in the United States lived more than 50 miles from a multidisciplinary clinic and nearly 25 percent were living more than 100 miles from a multidisciplinary clinic (Horton et al., 2018). However, in 2013,

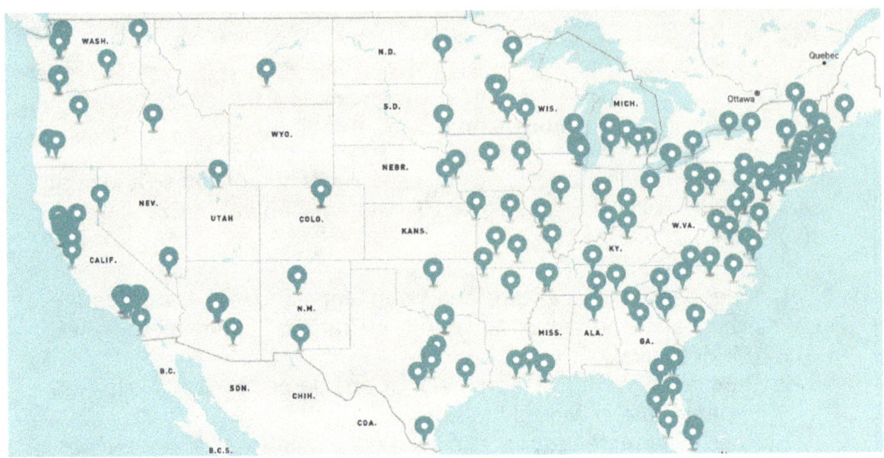

FIGURE 4-1 ALS clinic map.
SOURCE: I AM ALS, 2024.

there were only 72 multidisciplinary clinics across the country, including those operated by ALSA, MDA, and the Les Turner ALS Foundation (Horton et al., 2018). Today, ALSA alone has 89 Certified Treatment Centers of Excellence, which is its highest designation. Nevertheless, the literature reveals significant use of telehealth by people living with ALS, suggesting substantial demand for multidisciplinary care outside their range of travel (Haulman et al., 2020; Helleman et al., 2020). One result of a lack of universal access to a multidisciplinary clinic is that the average time from symptom onset to a patient's first appointment at a multidisciplinary clinic in the United States is 19 months (Galvin et al., 2015).

Cost is another significant barrier to accessing multidisciplinary care, estimated at $70,000 to $180,000 annually for each person living with ALS in the United States (Gladman and Zinman, 2015; Obermann and Lyon, 2015). As discussed in Chapter 3, people living with ALS bear much of this cost out of pocket. Other cost-related issues include the varying acceptability of insurance at each clinic, as well as systems of referral and prior authorization. Barriers related to distance and cost are further compounded by marginalization across racial, ethnic, and income-related lines.

The limited data regarding the use and access to multidisciplinary care in the United States suggest that many people with ALS cannot access multidisciplinary clinics or face significant barriers such as travel and cost. Thus, it is critical to improve access to multidisciplinary care so every person with ALS can receive state-of-the-art, evidence-based care without an undue burden from travel or cost.

Variation in Multidisciplinary ALS Care Teams

The structure of multidisciplinary ALS clinics varies widely in terms of their size and the scope of care they provide. In addition, ALS clinic team requirements and expectations vary across VA, ALSA, and MDA clinics (see Table 4-1). The ALS multidisciplinary care team can vary depending on whether team members are based in the multidisciplinary clinic or whether they are part of the external network of medical specialists, in-patient or nursing care institutions, home health agencies, not-for-profit ALS groups, and other DME experts from whom ALS individuals and families may receive care.

TABLE 4-1 ALS Clinic Team Requirements and Expectations Across VA, ALSA, and MDA Clinics

VA Interdisciplinary ALS Care Teams	ALSA-Certified Multidisciplinary Clinics	MDA Certified Clinics
Require, at a minimum: • ALS team physician • Coordinator • Social worker • Speech language pathologist • Physical therapist • Occupational therapist • Respiratory therapist • Dietician Other team members may include a primary care provider, home-based primary care team staff member, physiatrist, therapeutic recreational specialist, assistive technology specialist, kinesiotherapist, clinical pharmacist, psychologist, pulmonologist, gastroenterologist, palliative medicine/hospice care specialist, or chaplain.	Clinics follow the American Academy of Neurology Clinical Practice Guidelines, which lists the following as key members of the multidisciplinary team: • Physician • Physical therapist • Occupational therapist • Speech pathologist • Dietitian • Social worker • Respiratory therapist • Nurse case manager No care team members are explicitly required under any guidance the committee found. Other professionals mentioned in ALSA multidisciplinary care documents include ALS and neuromuscular neurologists, mental health professionals, and an ALSA liaison. Many ALSA clinics also employ a clinical coordinator, who may serve in another role on the multidisciplinary team and serves as the primary point person at the clinic.	May include on their care team: • MDA staff • Cardiologist • Dietitian/nutritionist • Genetic counselor • Neurologist • Nurse • Orthopedist • Physiatrist • Primary care physician • Psychiatrist • Psychologist • Pulmonologist • Respiratory therapist • Social worker • Speech/language pathologist No requirements are explicitly listed. Most MDA care centers are led by a neurologist or physiatrist. MDA care centers also include care center coordinators.

SOURCES: MDA, 2023; Miller et al., 2009; VHA, 2021.

Each ALS clinic in the United States today operates almost entirely on its own, with little connection to other ALS clinics. Clinic staff also vary in size and specialty. The committee was unable to find peer-reviewed literature discussing the staffing models at different clinics. However, the following breakdown reflects the committee's experience and information-gathering discussions:

- Smaller ALS clinics serving fewer than 100 people with ALS annually may have a core clinical team comprising an ALS specialist physician, a part-time physical therapist, and a part-time ALS nurse who staffs a half-day ALS clinic one or two times a month while performing other hospital and clinical duties during the remainder of the month.
- Larger ALS clinics serving from 100 to 1,000 people or more with ALS annually typically have a core clinic team comprising:
    - One to seven ALS specialists;
    - Up to six full-time or part-time ALS nurses;
    - Up to six full-time ALS nurse practitioners or other advanced practice providers;
    - Allied health clinicians, including one to four full-time or part-time ALS physical therapists, as many as two part-time ALS speech therapists and two part-time ALS occupational therapists; and
    - One to three full-time ALS patient service coordinators, up to six part-time ALS clinic coordinators for clinical outcomes collection, and one case manager or social worker.

If the resources are available, many larger clinics may have additional clinical staff such as electrophysiologists, geneticists and genetic counselors, respiratory therapists, palliative care specialists, pulmonologists, mental health professionals, interventional radiologists, care coordinators, house call nurses, and community health workers. These team members may be a direct part of the multidisciplinary ALS clinic infrastructure. Others may primarily provide care at another clinic within the same institution or system, while being connected to the multidisciplinary ALS clinic. The ALS specialist physicians staffing these clinics are generally neurologists with subspecialty training in neuromuscular disorders or neuropalliative care, or they may be physical medicine and rehabilitation specialists with training or experience in ALS.

The VA ALS Care System as a Potential Model
for Removing Barriers and Care Delays

The VA ALS system of care developed organically following the granting of service connection for ALS with clinics following the American Academy of Neurology clinical practice guidelines. In 2021, VA partnered with ALSA to increase the number of VA ALS clinics certified as Treatment Centers of Excellence.

VA's ALS specialty clinics provide multidisciplinary care to veterans with ALS, who account for more than 16 percent of individuals living with ALS (Valor Healthcare, n.d.). Based in part on a 2006 Institute of Medicine report, VA decided in 2008 that any veteran who develops ALS and served more than 90 days in any military branch with an honorable discharge is eligible for VA care as a 100 percent service-connected condition (IOM, 2006).[4] As a result, veterans with ALS and their families receive these benefits:

- All health care services, whether related to ALS or not;
- No copays for medical care, prescriptions, and DME;
- Power mobility, assistive technology, adaptive recreation, and respiratory equipment, with no limitations on when or how often equipment can be ordered;
- Monthly special disability compensation that ranges from approximately $4,000 to $9,000 per month;
- Paid home caregiver support, up to 65 percent of monthly skilled nursing facility costs;
- Special Adaptive Housing grant of more than $100,000 to cover modifications for home accessibility or to reduce mortgage and mortgage insurance payments;
- Adult day health and custodial care in the veteran's home or by a contracted skilled nursing facility or ventilator-capable skilled nursing facility;
- A grant of more than $24,000 toward purchasing a wheelchair-capable van or other adaptive vehicle;
- Transportation to and from medical appointments and lodging when necessary; and
- Enrollment in VA's Civilian Health and Medical Program, the federal health benefits program for family members of totally and permanently disabled veterans with a service-related disability.

A unique and important feature of the VA model versus non-VA ALS care (see Table 4-2) is that veterans with ALS are often spared the debilitating financial burdens related to receiving ongoing care, accessing pharmacological and nonpharmacological therapies, and maintaining DME. As discussed in Chapters 2 and 3, many people living with ALS face difficulties

---

[4]Presumptive Service Connection for Amyotrophic Lateral Sclerosis, CFR 38.3.318. https://www.ecfr.gov/current/title-38/chapter-I/part-3/subpart-A/subject-group-ECFR39056aee4e9ff13/section-3.318 (accessed May 10, 2024).

TABLE 4-2 Differences in VA Versus Non-VA ALS Care

Service	VA	Non-VA (Private Insurance, Medicare)
Pharmacological therapies	Consistent policy across VA centers; newly approved, expensive ALS drugs available based on prespecified criteria from clinical trials	More variability in coverage
Initiation of respiratory care	No restrictions	Requires forced vital capacity of less than 50 percent for noninvasive ventilation support
Durable medical equipment	No restrictions	Medicare: 1 wheelchair every 5 years
Acute in-patient rehabilitation	No absolute restrictions; admissions based upon medical judgment of physical medicine and rehabilitation physician	Medicare: 3-hour rule
Recreation therapy	No restrictions	Not widely available
Assistive technology	No restrictions	Not widely available
Driver's rehabilitation	No restrictions	Not widely available
Telehealth	No restrictions; VA clinicians authorized to provide telehealth care to any U.S. state[a]	Limitations on telehealth across state lines; allied health not always covered
Establishing care at more than one ALS center for different care needs	No restrictions; ALS patients can seek multidisciplinary ALS care at multiple locations within and outside of the VA system	Restrictions based on insurance network and state lines; for many payers, the frequency of ALS clinic follow-up visits cannot be less than 3 months apart
Care navigator services	Every person with ALS has a designated ALS coordinator for coordinating care within and outside VA ALS clinics (VHA Directive 1101.07)	Not available for most payer plans or ALS clinics
Research	No designated funding for research infrastructure to support clinical trials	Varied capabilities for research across clinics[b]
Expanded access to investigational therapeutics	Limited	Varied across clinics
Geographic distribution of care delivery centers	Limited; many patients travel several hours to reach an ALS clinic	Limited; many patients travel several hours to reach an ALS clinic

[a] 38 CFR § 17.417

[b] Many centers varyingly offer clinical trials, expanded access programs, registry enrollment, natural history studies, and clinical biomarker research. There is a growing number of centers that are connected to central or smart Institutional Review Boards, have reliance agreements in place facilitating participation in multisite research operations, and have established clinical research infrastructure and processes. One example is the 74-site Healey ALS platform trial.

obtaining prior authorization and financial burdens from early and continued access to specialist consultations, medications, therapies, and care services.

INTEGRATING CLINICAL RESEARCH INTO THE ALS CARE DELIVERY NETWORK

Over the past decade, ALS drug development in the United States and globally has expanded rapidly, indicating industry interest in this disease. As of 2020, there were at least 120 experimental therapeutics and gene therapies in active ALS clinical trials with a global market estimated to reach $1.02 billion by 2032 (GlobalData, 2021; Market.US, 2023). Despite this, in the committee's discussions with ALS clinical trialists, they heard that the difficulty of recruiting enough interested and willing people with ALS to a clinical trial slows the drug development process. The committee also heard that there are individuals with ALS interested in participating in clinical trials, but the restrictive inclusion criteria intended to enhance the scientific validity of the study also preclude some people with ALS from participating. Input from individuals with ALS and at-risk genetic carriers revealed multiple reasons they would want to participate in clinical trials. These include:

- Potentially receiving a new drug or intervention that is not available outside of a clinical trial;
- Contributing to drug development and science to help others who have or will develop ALS;
- Doing one's part as a research participant when it is estimated that only 10 percent of people with ALS participate in clinical trials;
- Providing hope and purpose during a difficult disease course;
- Providing a sense of control by taking a more active role in one's health care;
- Demonstrating to worried family that you are doing everything possible to improve your chance of survival;
- Setting an example for others of how to react to a life-altering illness;
- Creating more opportunities to learn about one's own illness status and progress, and potentially receive more observations and data points to follow;
- Learning about potential new treatments one may have an opportunity to take in the future; and
- Because it feels good to be part of research to find new treatments.

Overall, studies have shown that less than 10 percent of people with ALS participate in clinical trials and research, in contrast to other rare diseases such as pediatric cancer, which has a 60 percent participation rate (Bedlack et al., 2008; Gelijns and Gabriel, 2012; Mehta et al., 2021). A 2019 survey found that while 78 percent of individuals living with ALS would participate in clinical trials, only 20 percent knew a great deal about ALS clinical trials. Of those who had not participated in a clinical trial, 17 percent were unaware of any trials and 13 percent did not know how to find information about trials (Ipsos, 2019). The same survey reported that nearly 40 percent knew someone who could not afford to participate in a clinical trial because of travel costs, 25 percent feared participating, and nearly 75 percent were more likely to consider participating if they had a patient navigator or advocate at their primary hospital. In addition, there are racial and ethnic disparities in trial access and participation; less than 10 percent of ALS research participants are from underrepresented, minoritized populations (Raymond et al., 2019). Given these statistics, it would behoove the ALS community to make all individuals with ALS and at-risk genetic carriers aware of clinical trial opportunities early and universally and to encourage them to take advantage of the opportunity to participate in clinical trials.

One proven approach to increase clinical trial enrollment of a more diverse patient group is to create a coordinated, integrated network of sites, which would both provide clinical care for individuals with ALS and serve as a clinical trial and research network. Pediatric oncology, cancer, and cystic fibrosis models have shown that integrating research with clinical care and allowing every patient to participate in clinical trials—without increasing their travel or cost burden—accelerates progress, largely by increasing enrollment (Gelijns and Gabriel, 2012; Woodcock et al., 2021). The committee proposes a similar framework of integrating clinical trials into a clinical care network to address the current knowledge gap in ALS patients about clinical trials. While scientific breakthroughs and innovative trial designs are important, increasing trial participation and equity in access are equally important to accelerate ALS therapeutic development.

Another major obstacle to ALS trial and research participation is a narrow window of eligibility; many patients are diagnosed and placed on treatment late, at which point they fail to meet inclusion criteria, leading to missed opportunities. Many recent and ongoing clinical trials prioritize enrollment of early ALS patients within 18 months from symptom onset and that have been on standard-of-care medications for a few months before participation (Albanese et al., 2022; Paganoni et al., 2021).

Aside from the lack of patient knowledge of trials and diagnostic delay, a few other reasons might account for low enrollment in ALS clinical trials, including:

- As the number of FDA-approved ALS treatments expands, the existing therapeutic regimen can become more demanding for patients, making it more difficult to manage existing treatments and participate in clinical trials for new drugs.

- Clinical trials may be unattractive to individuals living with ALS because of the possibility of receiving a placebo instead of the study intervention, travel time to the trial site, financial burdens, and painful procedures or drug administration.
- Patients may distrust the medical system because of historic mistreatment and ongoing discrimination and inequities.

BUILDING THE IDEAL ALS CARE DELIVERY SYSTEM

Making ALS a livable disease requires diagnosing individuals earlier, in order to initiate evidence-based multidisciplinary care by ALS specialists immediately and continuously. At the same time, the progressive nature of the disease often makes travel difficult. Therefore, to facilitate continuous multidisciplinary care and support throughout their illness, individuals living with ALS will need access to centers at geographically accessible locations within their communities. However, it is not feasible to establish new stand-alone and dedicated multidisciplinary ALS centers to serve every person with ALS immediately near their home given resource and workforce restraints. However, existing resources may be leveraged and expanded to deliver care to more people with ALS closer to their homes. Thus, to increase access to state-of-the-art care and clinical research for every person with ALS, the committee recommends that a new ALS care system be established:

Recommendation 4-1: Build an inclusive and integrated ALS multidisciplinary care and research system.

The Centers for Medicare & Medicaid Services and the National Institute of Neurological Disorders and Stroke, in partnership with current ALS multidisciplinary care clinic system leaders (e.g., U.S. Department of Veterans Affairs, ALS Association, Muscular Dystrophy Association), and community-based providers should build an inclusive and integrated multidisciplinary care and research system for people living with ALS. This network should consist of:
   a. Community-Based ALS Centers,
   b. Regional ALS Centers, and
   c. Comprehensive ALS Care and Research Centers.

This new system, modeled after "hub-and-spoke" systems of care and research for cancer and stroke, is designed to fill gaps in access to ALS care and research across the United States. The Comprehensive ALS Care and Research Centers will serve as "hubs," centralizing oversight, while the Community-Based ALS Care Centers and Regional ALS Centers will serve as "spokes" (see Figure 4-2).

Each care setting in the network should provide defined clinical care services, enrollment in the National ALS Registry, and access to clinical research. They will also be accountable for achieving quality metrics. Their accreditation would be based on these capabilities and metrics, pursuant to nationally recognized quality metrics like those set and revised by the American Academy of Neurologists (AAN). This reimagined ALS care system will build on and strengthen the preexisting ALSA- and MDA-certified multidisciplinary clinic systems, centralizing oversight to ensure care quality, provide additional infrastructures to collect population health data (see Chapter 6), and coordinate care across levels.

Building on current ALS clinic accreditation programs, this system will bring in new clinics to increase the number of clinics providing this high-quality care. This includes community neurologists, private and group practices, as well as clinics that provide multidisciplinary care for neurological diseases other than ALS. Innovative approaches to bringing care to people with ALS will also be encouraged; examples may include expanded telehealth services, house call visits, and travel or satellite clinics. By bringing in this wide variety of care settings, areas without a large number of people with ALS will still have clinics available.

This system will also enhance participation in clinical research. As "hubs," Comprehensive ALS Care and Research Centers will be expected to have substantial breadth and depth of ALS research, including preclinical, clinical, preventive, and population-based research. Regional and even community-based centers without the capacity to lead major clinical research will be able to provide people with ALS access to research through their connections to hubs. In this way, people with ALS will have better access to clinical trials, natural history studies, and other research even if they are not receiving care at a Comprehensive ALS Center. All levels of care will facilitate enrollment in a more comprehensive National ALS Registry, as described in Chapter 6.

Hubs will also support spoke centers in several additional ways, increasing the quality of ALS diagnosis, care, and research across wide geographic areas. Most directly, hub centers will complement services provided by regional and community-based ALS centers as necessary. This will include consultation for complex care or diagnostic needs, as well as connecting people with ALS to comprehensive centers via telehealth. Hub centers will provide a full spectrum of diagnostic and referral services for primary care providers, community neurologists, and other specialists. Hubs will also be responsible for developing, promoting, and sharing professional education resources, as well as spearheading community outreach initiatives.

Establishing this reimagined system will require partnerships across the government (i.e., National Institutes of Health [NIH]/National Institute of

Neurological Diseases and Stroke [NINDS], Centers for Medicare & Medicaid Services [CMS]), current ALS multidisciplinary clinic system leaders (i.e., ALSA, MDA), home health agencies, community-based providers, and local community support organizations to (1) create new public–private partnerships and community-based connections, and (2) provide financial incentives to bring more community-based practitioners under the umbrella of this integrated hub-and-spoke model of ALS care. The roles of each type of clinic are described below.

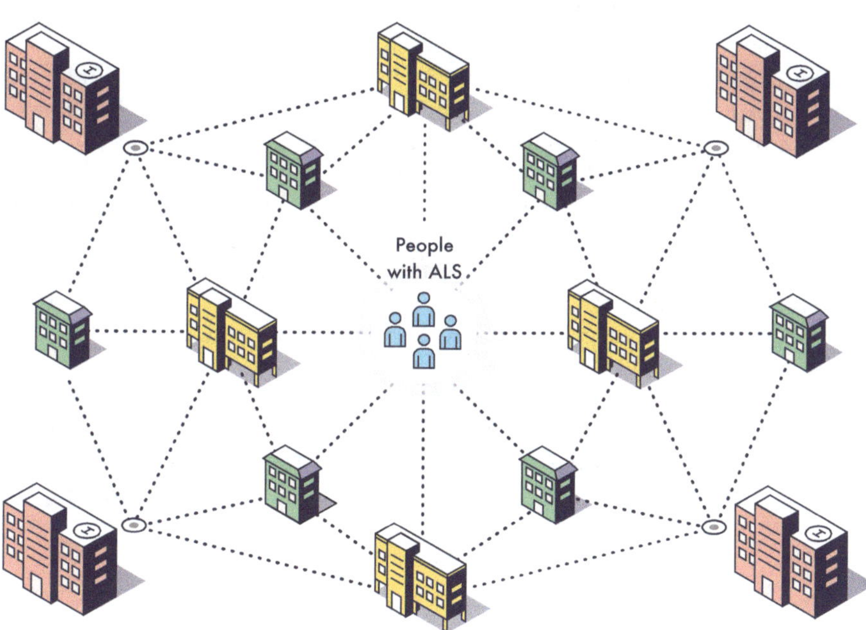

FIGURE 4-2 A reimagined ALS hub-and-spoke care system to increase access to multidisciplinary care.

Community-Based ALS Care Centers

Establishing a larger number of local, certified community-based multidisciplinary ALS care centers will facilitate access to high-quality routine care without requiring people with ALS to travel great distances. These centers may not have the same resources or organization as a dedicated ALS multidisciplinary clinic. They may instead be independent ALS clinics, other multidisciplinary neurological clinics, integrated care networks of various specialists, solo or group neurology practices, or even certain VA clinics. However, they will still be accountable for providing multidisciplinary ALS care adhering to the latest quality metrics and practice standards. These clinics will primarily provide post-diagnosis, routine follow-up care following a care plan formulated by a Comprehensive ALS Care and Research Center or Regional ALS Center (discussed below). Importantly, all clinical staff at these credentialed community-based centers would be trained in standard ALS clinical outcomes and monitoring. This training is already available and can be expanded; examples include trainings developed by the Northeast ALS Consortium (NEALS) Outcome Center, educational webinars, and continuing medical education (CME) programs.

Community-Based ALS Care Centers may lack the infrastructure locally to lead clinical research efforts. However, persons living with ALS receiving care would still be able to participate in clinical research through their community clinic, since community clinics will be integrated with regional and comprehensive clinics. In that way, community-based clinics would be able to recruit a more diverse population, increasing representation in research and reducing inequities. Furthermore, community-based clinic staff would coordinate with home health providers to meet the out-of-clinic needs of people with ALS and their families. These clinics would also have the capacity to engage at-risk ALS genetic carriers and facilitate their access to ALS registries.

Therefore, in this new, integrated model, people with ALS who live farther from a Comprehensive or Regional ALS Center may visit Community-Based ALS Care Centers for services such as:

- Initial diagnosis, with referral or consultation to other ALS centers available for second opinions;
- Day-to-day, routine follow-up care post-diagnosis, adhering to AAN quality metrics and practice standards;
- Connection to community-based primary care and support agencies, telehealth, home health, palliative and hospice agencies, and DME companies;
- Participation in research, such as clinical trials and natural history studies; and
- Referral to other local specialists or community-based organizations for further support.

Certified community-based ALS care clinics could include current ALSA- or MDA-affiliated clinics, along with new entities brought on board to increase access to care throughout the country. For example, existing multidisciplinary centers catering to other neuromuscular or neurological disorders, such as multiple sclerosis, muscular dystrophy, Charcot-Marie-Tooth disease, spinal muscular atrophy, Huntington's disease, Parkinson's disease, or dementia, that may not be dedicated ALS clinics as part of current ALSA, MDA, or VA systems but could enter the new integrated care and research system and be accredited to treat ALS. Using an existing multidisciplinary clinic staffing infrastructure will be especially critical in geographic areas where there are fewer people living with ALS—or clinicians with knowledge about ALS—to develop and sustain a dedicated ALS clinic.

New community-based ALS clinics could be incentivized to care for people living with ALS via new reimbursement models. For instance, a group of ALS clinicians, specialists, and allied health professionals, including home-based palliative and home health care professionals within a community, may organize into an integrated care network and receive accreditation to deliver ALS multidisciplinary care. By incentivizing specialists who already practice in an area to create an integrated care network, commit to delivering high-quality ALS multidisciplinary care, and meet all other accreditation requirements, multidisciplinary care can still be delivered in less-resourced settings or in those with fewer people with ALS. In summary, certified community-based ALS care clinics would provide localized multidisciplinary care currently missing in the ALS care system. Staff at these clinics would be trained in ALS-specific clinical outcomes, quality metrics, other practice standards, and the latest updates in care by CME courses. Certified community-based ALS care clinics would also offer ALSA- or MDA-led education on ALS awareness.

Regional ALS Centers

Larger multidisciplinary clinics dedicated to ALS would be designated as Regional ALS Centers. While Community-Based ALS Care Centers would be responsible for ongoing management of routine care, they may not have the capacity for more complex, surgical, or specialized care needs. Regional ALS Centers would have the staffing and facilities necessary to provide such care, and as a result, many would be at larger hospitals. Like the other two levels, such centers would provide high-quality, post-ALS diagnosis multidisciplinary care according to AAN quality metrics; they would also provide a wider range of diagnostic and care services than community-based centers.

Nevertheless, Regional ALS Centers may not have the capacity to provide all ALS diagnosis or complex multispecialty care and services, such as those related to complex imaging, genetic testing, or counseling. They would, however, be able to provide specialty care and support services, while referring to or consulting Comprehensive ALS Care and Research Centers as needed. This integration would allow for telehealth consults with Comprehensive ALS Care and Research Centers for second opinions or complex care needs. This is similar to the American Heart Association and American Stroke Association's comprehensive stroke centers, which provide telehealth-based second opinions to smaller stroke centers.

Unlike the Comprehensive ALS Care and Research Centers discussed next, Regional ALS Centers may not have the capacity to coordinate or lead cutting-edge ALS clinical research, or to secure federal funding for preclinical research. This builds on the preexisting ALSA model of multidisciplinary care, which primarily differentiates between levels based on whether research is offered. Like all clinics in this reimagined integrated care and research system, Regional ALS Centers would offer the opportunity to participate in clinical trials or expanded access programs, enroll people with ALS in a more comprehensive National ALS Registry or natural history studies, and report on quality and population health outcomes.

Specialty services delivered by Regional ALS Centers may include:

- Diagnostic assessment and confirmation
- Specialized follow-up care needs such as:
  o Pulmonary care,
  o Tracheostomy or ventilation support,
  o Evaluation for specialized DME such as eye-tracking communication devices,
  o Medically complex cases requiring surgical procedures or post-procedural intensive care, and
  o Augmented communication and technological care services
- Support for insurance approval of standard-of-care therapies

Comprehensive ALS Care and Research Centers

Comprehensive ALS Care and Research Centers, like all clinics in this model, would provide high-quality multidisciplinary care based on the latest practice standards, facilitate access to research, and enroll people with ALS into the National ALS Registry. Beyond that, however, they would also serve as hubs that would:

- Actively conduct clinical trials and clinical research projects.
- Provide the research community with centralized imaging, biofluid and tissue biorepositories, and registry services.

- Engage genetic carriers and facilitate access to ALS research opportunities for genetic carriers.
- Train and develop the ALS workforce.

To serve as a hub and facilitate access to cutting-edge services for every ALS patient, clinicians at Comprehensive ALS Care and Research Centers should be allowed to provide consultations, second opinions, and other care services via telehealth without state line restrictions to patients receiving care at regional and community centers and their physicians. This would align with the current VA ALS system of care, which currently universally permits interstate telehealth within the Veterans Health Administration.[5] The committee recognizes that telehealth policies are complex, vary across states, and are constantly evolving. Telehealth capabilities that cross states lines to allow ALS centers to coordinate and provide a high level of care to all persons with ALS would improve the success of the newly integrated system. VA is already allowed to use telehealth to serve veterans with ALS, and the committee believes persons with ALS who receive care outside the VA system also deserve access to the benefits of telehealth.

Care Quality Metrics

Like all accredited clinics, Comprehensive ALS Care and Research Centers will provide care following AAN quality metrics,[6] along with routinely offered ALS diagnostic, therapeutic, and, when approved for future clinical practice, preventive services. These services would include standard-of-care treatments and procedures, electromyogram and nerve conduction studies, genetic testing and counseling, biofluid or neuroimaging biomarker testing if approved for future clinical practice, functional rating scales, and respiratory tests. As the literature develops and the standard of care continues to advance, such as with ongoing revisions to the AAN guidelines, quality metrics may continue to change as well. Certified raters would regularly assess these and other clinical outcome measures to monitor disease progression and other specialty services at their institution, such as pulmonology, physical medicine and rehabilitation, urology, psychology or psychiatry, and interventional radiology.

Clinical Research Capabilities and Expectations

Since clinical research drives innovation and therapeutic discoveries for ALS, Comprehensive ALS Care and Research Centers will need to integrate clinical research into clinical care, contributing to population

---

[5] 38 CFR § 17.417.

[6] Available at https://www.aan.com/practice/neuromuscular-quality-measures (accessed June 10, 2024).

health outcomes research and care delivery research. These centers will need to engage in high-volume natural history, registry, or other biomarker research; participate in presymptomatic gene carrier research; participate in a clinical research consortium or care delivery network; and offer clinical trials or expanded access protocols. To facilitate care coordination and research recruitment, these centers must have at least one full-time patient research and care navigator on staff.

Like the National Cancer Institute model of Comprehensive Cancer Centers, Comprehensive ALS Care and Research Centers would be incentivized to lead community outreach and engagement efforts and coordinate with Regional ALS Centers and Community-Based ALS Care Clinics to increase access among individuals from underserved populations and to ensure continuity of care, even in later disease stages or when a patient can no longer travel. As discussed in greater detail later in this chapter, such efforts may include setting up community engagement and advisory committees comprising community-based ALS and caregiver members, non-profit organizations and foundations, primary care physicians, and home health agencies to understand the changing care needs and barriers to health care use and participation in the local community.

Comprehensive ALS Care and Research Centers could also pilot or expand creative care delivery programs such as ALS house call nursing programs, ALS multidisciplinary mobile clinics, travel satellite clinics, and medical home programs, which are active in some U.S. regions. Such programs could bring care closer to the homes of persons living with ALS to reduce travel burden, particularly during the later disease stages. Box 4-2 describes the specialty care medical home as a potential model for coordinating community-based multidisciplinary care for ALS.

Integration Across Levels

People with ALS may enter this new integrated care and research system in a variety of ways. Some people with ALS see an ALS specialist relatively early, or they may see clinicians at hospitals that have Comprehensive ALS Care and Research Centers or Regional ALS Centers. Others may initially see their primary care physician or non-ALS specialists. A person suspected to have ALS will be referred to the nearest comprehensive or regional center for diagnostic confirmation, formulation of a multidisciplinary care plan, and a discussion of opportunities to participate in research. For complex scenarios, they may also use telehealth for remote second opinions with Comprehensive ALS Care and Research Centers. Telehealth will also be available for second opinions and referrals throughout all levels of the system.

BOX 4-2
**Specialty Care Medical Home: A Model for Coordinating
Community-Based Multidisciplinary Care for ALS**

In a traditional medical home model, a primary care practice is accountable for meeting the majority of each patient's physical and mental health care needs. Rather than being centered around a primary care practice, the Specialty Care Medical Home model centers care around neurologists and related professionals while continuing to coordinate care with a patient's primary care provider. NeurAbilities Healthcare, the model's developer, provides outpatient, ambulatory care within office, home, school, and community-based venues, as well as via telemedicine. Its integrated multidisciplinary and interdisciplinary clinical team consists of neurologists, child neurologists, developmental-behavioral pediatricians, medical geneticists, advanced practice providers, neuropsychologists, clinical psychologists, board-certified behavior analysts, registered behavior technicians, licensed professional counselors, cognitive behavioral therapists, creative arts therapists, neurotechnologists, and medical assistants. The Clinical Research Center of New Jersey provides patients access to industry-sponsored clinical trials and physician-initiated research.

SOURCE: Mintzi, 2022.

The comprehensive or regional ALS center would continue to provide follow-up specialist appointments for continuity of care or complication management as necessary. Day-to-day, routine follow-up care would be managed by the nearest available multidisciplinary center (whether comprehensive, regional, or community-based). All levels will have the capacity to deliver this care; by integrating more ALS centers, especially Community-Based ALS Care Centers, into the system, more people with ALS will have standard of care treatments available to them.

ALS research is also integrated into this reimagined system. Regardless of what type of clinic a person with ALS attends for their routine care, they will always have access to clinical research due to the integrated nature of the system. All center types in this new integrated care and research system will be incentivized to enroll and retain all people with ALS in the National ALS Registry, as proposed in Chapter 6, for population health monitoring.

How the Integrated ALS Care and Research Model Should Work

The above model will create a highly integrated system of care that should more easily reach underrepresented and underserved ALS patients and those living in remote areas of the United States and all U.S. territories and improve the current system of care for individuals living with ALS (see Table 4-3). Today, many non-ALS-trained neurologists provide care to ALS patients in general neurology or general neuromuscular clinics, which, under the new recommended model, could be integrated into the new ALS care system under the guidance of the comprehensive ALS centers. This would expand the number of general neurology and neuromuscular clinics within the ALS care and research system, enhancing access to care and reducing the time to diagnosis.

The newly networked community-based or regional clinic would be responsible for measuring and improving diagnostic timelines within its geographic area. A designated person or team would coordinate with the hub and take action to reduce delays in diagnosis. The designated diagnostic person or team could work proactively with local Federally Qualified Health Centers (FQHCs) and local practices such as sports rehabilitation or general neurology clinics to educate non-ALS specialists on how to identify possible ALS symptoms and instruct them on the referral process to the local ALS specialist. The Comprehensive ALS Care and Research Centers coordinating the local diagnostic teams would be adequately reimbursed to dedicate time and attention identifying people who may have ALS and educating local providers, but this expense is necessary to improve the diagnosis process.

The NINDS Access for All in ALS (ALL ALS) research consortium and network of sites, initiated in 2023, could serve as a foundation on which to build the ideal ALS care network. Currently, the ALL ALS consortium, funded under the Accelerating Access to Critical Therapies for ALS Act,[7] primarily collects natural history, clinical, biomarker, and imaging data, along with autopsy tissue, from several thousand people with ALS and deposits them in central data banks and biological specimen banks for future research. However, the committee envisions this consortium's network could be developed or expanded to meet the goals of the proposed care delivery network, as successfully achieved by several National Cancer Institute–funded care delivery networks.

---

[7]Accelerating Access to Critical Therapies for ALS Act, Public Law 117-79.

TABLE 4-3 Comparing the Current ALS Clinical Care and Research System to the Committee's Proposal for an Integrated ALS Care and Research System

	Current Clinical System and Research System	Proposed Integrated Care and Research System
Number of individuals living with ALS served	Unknown but one estimate is that, at best, half of individuals living with ALS receive care at multidisciplinary clinics.[a]	All individuals living with ALS are served through the proliferation of community-based centers that offer standard of care integrated into a broader network of ALS centers.
At-risk genetic carriers	At-risk genetic carriers have limited access to multidisciplinary clinics.	All interested at-risk genetic carriers will have access to at-risk genetic carrier resources and help routing to natural history studies, which include care and interventions, via the community, regional, or comprehensive centers. Tools will be available for primary care providers to use for individuals at genetic risk of ALS.
Racial equity	Measures of equity are uncertain or not measured.	Centers will be accountable for measuring and addressing access to diagnosis and care in their geographic area.
Time to diagnosis	Delays of 10 to 19 months from first symptom to diagnosis exist. Black individuals wait 50 percent longer than White patients to receive a diagnosis.	Centers will be accountable for reducing diagnostic delays in their geographic area. This could be via a team or an individual with the specific responsibility of educating local providers about ALS, how to recognize possible symptoms, and refer. Better education for first-line physicians and offering diagnostic and referral tools to better and more quickly recognize ALS. For example, not "waiting and watching" but using tools such as thinkALS (ALSA, 2024).
Innovation	Varied, dependent on individual center resources.	Centers would be networked and share best practices and collaborate on new innovations (e.g., consider hiring former ALS caregivers to be community health workers and train current caregivers).

[a] In an October 18, 2023, letter to the committee from the ALS Association, it is stated: "Although multidisciplinary ALS care can add nine months of life, it is woefully underfunded and often difficult to deliver. Only about half the people served at ALSA Certified Treatment Centers of Excellence receive this well-established, evidence-based standard of care."

SOURCES: ALSA, 2024; Chen et al., 2023; Falcão de Campos et al., 2022; Galvin et al., 2015; Gwathmey et al., 2023a; Matharan et al., 2020; Richards et al., 2021.

ALS CARE SYSTEM CHALLENGES

The current ALS care system faces several challenges in providing timely and equitable access to high-quality multidisciplinary care for all people living with ALS. Among the most significant is the common delay in diagnosis (see Chapter 2), which averages 7 to 10 months for bulbar-onset ALS and 10 to 22 months for limb-onset ALS (Gwathmey et al., 2023b). While ALS remains invariably fatal, advances in therapeutic development and clinical research will likely prolong the lifespan and improve quality of life for people living with ALS. Given that prompt and early initiation of multidisciplinary care and medications improve outcomes, delays in diagnosis and treatment can significantly affect the course of the disease. Unacceptable delays result largely from delays in referral to an ALS specialist because the primary care physician did not recognize the ALS symptoms, referrals to one or more specialists other than a neurologist, and misdiagnosis, including by a general neurologist (Goyal et al., 2023; Matharan et al., 2020; Morren et al., 2023; Richards et al., 2021). Other factors delaying prompt diagnosis include age of onset—people with ALS older than 60 years of age are more likely to be initially misdiagnosed than are younger people with ALS (Belsh and Schiffman, 1996)—and neurological comorbidities (Mitchell et al., 2010; Palese et al., 2019). Moreover, coordination is lacking between general neurologists, who may only see a few people living with ALS each year, and ALS specialists.

Once a person with ALS is diagnosed, there is also variation across clinics in the quality and consistency of care they receive, including prescribing of standard-of-care therapeutics, use of noninvasive ventilation, use of off-label supplements and medications, clinical trial participation, and access to clinical trials (Chiò et al., 2011; Hogden and Crook, 2017; Katyal and Govindarajan, 2017; Skulstad Johanson et al., 2022; Thakore et al., 2019). Some ALS multidisciplinary clinics may not prescribe certain medications approved by the U.S. Food and Drug Administration because of perceived insufficient benefits, or offer genetic testing or counseling, evaluate voice or message banking, provide speech-generating devices, or offer the palliative care or hospice services as recommended (Fahrner-Scott et al., 2022).

Moreover, challenges exist from low clinic capacity and lack of training and growth opportunities for ALS specialists and the health care workforce. In addition to ALS specialists, pulmonologists, who provide critical life-extending respiratory care to people with ALS, are in limited supply, creating few opportunities for new consults (Ackrivo, 2023; Hansen-Flaschen, 2021). Access to essential home health aides and home care services are limited resulting from gross underpayment for hourly paid workers.

Administrative burden and insurance conflicts also affect many ALS multidisciplinary clinics and the individuals they serve. Clinic staff spend hours filling out paperwork, seeking prior authorization, calling insurers and pharmacies, appealing denials, and fielding phone calls from people living with ALS and their families, which can delay or prevent using potentially effective therapies and engender patient dissatisfaction. This current inefficient system hinders ALS clinics from meeting the needs of people they are treating for ALS, slows their ability to serve new people with ALS, and results in redundancies that are a waste of time and money.

If the status quo of the current care system continues, increased demand from a growing ALS prevalence, both from more diagnosed individuals and people living longer with ALS, will worsen the existing inequities in access to multidisciplinary care. Therefore, as earlier diagnosis and therapeutic regimens improve, new ALS care delivery systems will need to be sufficiently coordinated and nimble to meet the evolving needs of individuals living with ALS. Furthermore, new ALS care standardization will reduce redundancies, facilitate care from physicians with experience treating individuals with ALS, and provide the latest evidence-based care. By integrating the new ALS care delivery and research systems as this chapter recommends, more people living with ALS will have access to high-quality care.

Meeting the Equity Challenge

Many people with ALS in historically marginalized and underserved communities do not have early or consistent access to multidisciplinary ALS centers and care. For example, the time it takes a Black individual with ALS to receive a diagnosis can be more than 50 percent longer than a White individual (Chen et al., 2023; Gwathmey et al., 2023a). This is despite the fact that Black people living with ALS were, in one study, found to live closer to a multidisciplinary center than White people living with ALS (Horton et al., 2018). Black people living with ALS are also often more advanced in their disease and disability at the time of diagnosis (Richards, 2020). Providers' implicit biases, structural racism, and patient distrust, disinterest, or fear of seeking medical attention are also sources of this racial disparity (Carter, 2021, 2022; Casey, 2023; Chen et al., 2023). The disparity in diagnosis time is also affected by the type of clinician people with ALS may visit initially to seek care. As discussed earlier, community-based clinicians without specific training or ALS experience may be less aware of the range of early-stage ALS signs. Efforts to improve health outcomes and reduce disparities for people with ALS will ideally move away from "cultural competency" education to "structural competency" and an understanding of the way social and economic forces influence health outcomes at levels above individual physician–patient interactions (Metzl and Hansen, 2014).

Significant racial inequities exist in the U.S. health care system overall—Black people and American Indians and Alaska Natives, for example, fared significantly worse across the majority of 30 measures of health status and health outcomes between 2019 and 2021 (Hill et al., 2023)—which the ALS care and research system exists within. However, it is worthwhile to pursue targeted approaches to improve racial equity in ALS, and the committee offers the following recommendation:

Recommendation 4-2: Improve racial and ethnic equity in the ALS care and research system.

ALS multidisciplinary clinics should partner with community members and community-serving organizations to pursue targeted approaches to understanding and improving racial and ethnic equity in ALS care and outcomes in their geographic area.

The committee believes there are several opportunities that ALS clinics, in partnership with entities that serve the local community such as FQHCs, should pursue, including the following:

- Create community-focused steering committees. Each Community-Based ALS Care Center, as recommended in this report, in the newly integrated ALS care and research system should include a steering committee that would include multiple community members—individuals living with ALS, former ALS caregivers, at-risk genetic carriers, and other ALS experts from diverse racial and ethnic backgrounds, including non-English speaking individuals, among others—to build a bridge to the community and help develop programs to bring people who might otherwise go unnoticed into the ALS system.
- Collect and analyze data on racial equity. ALS centers should be expected to measure and address racial equity. Local clinics should report on the unique factors contributing to diagnostic delays in their geographic area. This responsibility to their population could be tied to funding and be a condition of qualifying as an ALS center.
- Adopt antiracism and implicit bias training as an expected and regular part of training. Each Comprehensive ALS Care and Research Center should lead antiracism and implicit bias training for center staff and clinicians that is not a one-time exercise but a regular part of training. Training would include developing an understanding of disparities in ALS, the social and structural determinants of health, and what it looks like to provide good care to diverse and historically underrepresented populations.

Meeting the Challenge of Workforce Development and Education

Since ALS is a rare disease, a non-neuromuscular or non-ALS specialist neurologist may see only one or two people living with ALS in their clinical practice per year. It is even rarer for primary care physicians and other physicians, who may not recognize or consider ALS early in their diagnostic workup and differential diagnosis, but instead "wait and watch" until symptoms have progressed before they refer the person to specialized multidisciplinary clinic.

Training and education are needed to ensure that nonspecialist clinicians suspect and refer people who may have ALS, even if not fully meeting the traditional diagnostic criteria of ALS. Education and training should also include information on diseases that mimic ALS to reduce false positive referrals. The ALSA thinkALS tool is one approach to aid the non-ALS specialist clinician suspect ALS and reduce referral delays. Artificial intelligence tools could be developed that parse out pertinent clinical features from electronic health records during clinical consultation with a non-ALS physician, providing an alert about the possibility of ALS.

The projected increase in ALS prevalence will exacerbate the demand for the already limited number of ALS specialists and other clinician staff (Arthur et al., 2016; Miller et al., 2021). Optimal care for individuals living with ALS requires collaboration across multiple medical specialties, including neuromuscular neurology and physiatrists (McDonald and Fowler, 2012), but there are significant workforce limitations in neuromuscular specialists, affecting patient access to subspecialized care. For example, the American Board of Psychiatry and Neurology only issued 98 certifications for physicians specializing in neuromuscular medicine in 2022.[8]

There are gaps in clinician education about ALS diagnosis and the benefits of multidisciplinary care. For example, not all U.S. neurology residencies include ALS clinic rotations. In addition, there are only two to three dedicated ALS fellowships yearly to train the next generation of ALS clinicians, researchers, and clinical trialists. For example, the American Academy of Neurology offers one 2-year or 3-year clinical ALS research training grant awarded competitively to one clinician per year. Academic institutions may offer fellowships in neurodegenerative disorders that are limited and not linked to accreditation. Current NINDS career development, or K, awards focus mainly on helping postdoctoral fellows transition to independent investigators but are not set aside for a particular subspecialty.[9]

---

[8] Additional information is available at http://www.abpn.com/about/facts-and-statistics (accessed June 10, 2024).

[9] Additional information is available at https://www.ninds.nih.gov/funding/training-career-development/career-development-awards (accessed June 10, 2024).

CDC offers an ALS continuing education module for primary health providers and other health professionals.[10] It would be appropriate for every graduate medical, nursing, or physician assistant professional school to include an ALS module such as this in their curricula. Since most people with ALS die from respiratory failure, pulmonologists need training in the treatment and supportive care of people with ALS. Physiatrists, physical medicine, and rehabilitation specialists, palliative care clinicians, critical care specialists, emergency physicians, neurosurgeons, spine surgeons, and otolaryngologists would also benefit from ALS-specific training. Persons with ALS will need to receive care from other health professionals not specific to their ALS diagnosis, such as dentists, audiologists, and others, who would need to understand what ALS is and how the disease affects the person they are treating.

There is also a severe shortage of home health care workers. According to the Home Care Association of America, home health care providers turn away 25 percent of referred patients because of staff shortages (HCAA, 2023). Factors behind the shortage include low pay compared to other sectors, lack of opportunities for career advancement, dramatic slowdown in the flow of immigrants who usually account for most of this workforce, preference for part-time work to remain below income limits that qualify for public assistance benefits, and a first-year turnover rate of 64 percent (HCAA, 2023). As described in Chapters 2 and 3, persons with ALS have significant home health needs requiring a home health aide with knowledge of complex life-sustaining machinery, such as ventilators. It will be necessary to adequately compensate a trained home health workforce for their experience if ALS is to become a livable disease in the next 10 years.

The comprehensive ALS centers in the proposed network could serve as training facilities, tied to their certification, to develop yearlong clinician/clinical translational research fellowships and other short-term training programs. Doing so would create opportunities to train future ALS clinicians and clinical researchers, including physicians, advanced care practitioners, nurses, and allied health professionals. The newly proposed network would also be responsible for ongoing ALS education and training of the clinician and lay community. Funding for the new NINDS-funded research financing model recommended in this report could be earmarked for this training.

NINDS recently published a set of strategic priorities for the ALS community, including mechanisms to encourage pursual of ALS-related research and training (Koroshetz, 2023). NINDS, with the American Academy of Neurology and the Accreditation Council for Graduate Medical Education, could take steps to make the ALS specialty clinician, hybrid clinician,

---

[10]Additional information is available at https://www.cdc.gov/als/ce/Index.html (accessed June 10, 2024).

clinical trialist, or clinical researcher track a sustainable, adequately compensated, and more attractive career pathway for junior faculty entering the workforce to address the pending crisis regarding the shrinking ALS specialist workforce.

The proposed integrated ALS care and research model will only succeed if the workforce exists to meet the needs of persons living with ALS and their families. There is an urgent need for the public, private, and nonprofit sectors working in ALS to provide incentives and opportunities to recruit and retain the ALS workforce needed. This includes ALS specialists, clinical trialists, health service researchers, and the critically needed home health workforce with the skills to care for the complex needs of a person with ALS.

Meeting the Challenge of Payment and Reimbursement for ALS Multidisciplinary Care and Research

As discussed in Chapters 2 and 3, many persons with ALS and their families experience significant financial challenges. As noted above, multidisciplinary clinics also have significant financial challenges given the longer visits needed to diagnose and establish care for persons with ALS (Boylan et al., 2015; Paganoni et al., 2017). The traditional fee-for-service payment model fails to reimburse for more than 50 percent of the costs of an ALS multidisciplinary clinic visit (Boylan, 2015; Paganoni et al., 2017), so centers must seek philanthropic, foundational, and institutional resources to meet costs.

The current payer limitations of a fee-for-service payment model for evaluation and management encounters in ALS means that multidisciplinary ALS clinics are not reimbursed for many of the staff providing care during the ALS clinic visit, including physical therapists, occupational therapists, speech therapists, social workers, case managers, genetic counselors, ALS clinic nurses, certified ALS clinical outcomes monitoring services, and clinical research access coordinators. Under the fee-for-service model, institutions must absorb the indirect costs of the 4- to 5-hour long multidisciplinary visits since insurance reimbursements account for only 30- to 60-minute face-to-face time spent with the physician. There is also the financial burden arising from uncompensated time clinical staff spend coordinating the evaluation, insurance authorizations, coordinating care with home health and home hospice agencies, and communicating with people with ALS and their caregivers.

A 2015 report by the Massachusetts General Hospital ALS clinic, one of the largest U.S. ALS centers, showed that 409 unique people with ALS and 1,285 ambulatory office encounters averaged $580 in actual cost per patient per clinic visit. However, the insurance-billable encounter recouped only $263 per patient per clinic visit, leaving a $317 shortfall per patient per clinic visit (Paganoni et al., 2017). Nonprofit organizations, such as ALSA and MDA, and local nonprofits supporting single ALS centers, such as the Les Turner ALS Foundation in Chicago or the ALS Hope Foundation in Philadelphia, can offset some of these costs through semiregular, nonguaranteed funds. Moreover, donated funds may be insufficient to cover the shortfall; for example, ALSA contributes only $25,000 to each multidisciplinary clinic annually. Thus, for the most part, ALS clinics must self-support multidisciplinary clinic operational costs via the ALS clinic sundry funds, departmental, or institutional support, and philanthropic support.

Major health care institutions may support salary for one to two dedicated ALS registered nurses per ALS clinic based on insurance reimbursements. However, many major ALS centers see and provide care to 600 to more than 900 people with ALS annually and require as many as nine dedicated ALS registered nurses to adequately deliver high-quality nursing care. Because of staffing shortages at ALS clinics, the same nurses often also fulfill case management or social worker roles to coordinate care with local Visiting Nurse Association operations, palliative care teams, nursing homes, hospice, and insurance prior authorization and disability paperwork. Smaller ALS centers with limited financial resources to hire and support multiple ALS nurses refer their people with ALS to other larger centers, which may be as far as 100 miles away or across state lines.

Because of the continually changing care needs stemming from the progressive nature of ALS, care provided during clinic visits may not suffice. To provide optimal continuity of care, ALS nurses often spend multiple hours per week per patient answering patient or family phone calls or online portal messages related to clinical care, medication changes, or coordinating care with local primary care or other non-ALS care teams. Since there are no payment models or pathways for nurses to bill insurance for their services, they are not compensated for the vital services they provide to individuals living with ALS.

The current funding structure for ALS multidisciplinary clinics is not a sustainable model to provide high-quality care. A new model is necessary to make that care accessible to all people with ALS. Reimbursement policies need to promote the seamless delivery of clinical care and home-based services and equipment, including the use of telehealth to provide services across state lines. This is similar to what VA offers veterans with ALS.

The committee is aware of legislative efforts in Congress to create a supplemental, facility-based Medicare payment for ALS-related services at multidisciplinary clinics. Condition-specific reimbursement mechanisms have been implemented by CMS for end-stage renal disease, cancer, and other diseases. Such a model can be piloted by public actors such as the CMS Innovation Center or by private insurers.

The committee's broader vision for an integrated ALS care and research system includes a companion approach to reimbursement. Reimbursement policy can both increase the number of clinics caring for people with ALS and expand the geographic areas served by the ALS care and research system.

For example, large academic health systems could be incentivized to establish Comprehensive ALS Care and Research Centers, caring for more people with ALS and serving as research hubs. Increasing the number of these comprehensive ALS centers would establish a common infrastructure of trained and experienced health care personnel, which could also serve as centers for other neurological disorders that would benefit from similar multidisciplinary care, such as muscular dystrophies, inherited neuropathies, multiple sclerosis, Parkinson's disease, and dementia.

Similarly, clinics that do not serve substantial populations of people with ALS should be incentivized to become a Regional Multidisciplinary ALS Center or Community-Based Multidisciplinary ALS Care Clinic. For example, smaller clinics across multiple specialties could be incentivized to organize themselves into a disease-specific "pod" to provide multidisciplinary ALS care as an integrated care network. As discussed earlier, such a pod would obviate the need for creating an entirely new ALS clinic in an area where resource limitations would make that challenging. While they would serve other patients, they would be part of this new clinical care and research system as the equivalent to a single multidisciplinary clinic, with all the same accreditation standards.

This model would allow outreach, scalability, and the expansion of network sites, even to geographic areas with low ALS volume, while assuring access and connectivity for all persons with ALS to the specialized services they need and opportunities to participate in research more easily. Research center designation and reimbursement should track with the level of leadership and participation in the new integrated clinical care and research model.

Recommendation 4-3: Align reimbursement to achieve the goals of the ALS clinical care and research system.

The Centers for Medicare & Medicaid Services, private insurers, the National Institutes of Health, and the National Institute of Neurological Disorders and Stroke should align reimbursement and the goals of the new, inclusive, and integrated ALS clinical care and research system.

Value-Based Payments

In addition to greater overall reimbursement to accredited clinical programs that participate in the ALS research and clinical care system, value-based payments may help promote effective and high-quality care.[11] There are two options for creating value-based financing models to support the ALS care and research under the recommended integrated model.

The first option is for clinical programs to receive standard value-based payments for ALS multidisciplinary clinic encounters. In this model, clinics would bill for each evaluation and management encounter on a fee-for-service basis. Payments would then be adjusted for meeting key quality metrics, including measures of access and quality for care delivered in rural, low socioeconomic, and underrepresented and marginalized communities. In this model, reimbursements for surgical or medical procedures, such as per cutaneous gastrostomy, intrathecal or intravenous infusions, lumbar punctures, and electromyographies; inpatient hospitalization; emergency department costs; other outpatient specialist consultation referrals; and home health care costs provided within or outside the institution would be subject to standard fee-for-service or bundled payment models.

A second option is capitated payment, under which clinical programs would receive a global, value-based payment for all the care a person with ALS needs. For this payment, the clinical program would be responsible for providing individualized ALS care, regardless of how many evaluation and management encounters or home visit encounters that a person with ALS may need throughout the year.

Unlike adjustments to fee-for-service payments, global value-based payments can reflect the heterogeneity of ALS presentation and care. People with ALS would be able to receive care for their unique needs with fewer restrictions on timing, setting, or services available. As long as services are specified within the network beforehand, preapproval for specialty services (e.g., pulmonology, physiatry) would no longer be necessary, and delivery of support services (e.g., psychology, care navigation) can be supported. Under this model, insurance-based restrictions on the number of clinic visits a person with ALS may have within a certain length of time may also be removed. Finally, care across all three settings in the committee's proposed network would be coordinated, and home-based care could be further incentivized to bring care closer to people with ALS instead of relying on clinic visits alone.

Challenges to establishing capitated payments include setting the right level for people with different types of ALS and disease trajectories.

---

[11]Value-based capitation adds performance metrics to the capitation formula to ensure patients do not receive suboptimal care through under-utilization of health care services. Meeting or exceeding value-based performance metrics can be linked to financial rewards such a bonuses (Alguire, 2023).

Any definition of "value" in value-based care and associated reimbursement structures would need to be crafted carefully so as not to require patient improvement as part of the criteria. The heterogeneity in how ALS presents and progresses also may make it difficult to estimate per-person costs. For these reasons, caution in proceeding with fully capitated models too quickly is warranted.

Meeting the Challenge of Paying for Integrated ALS Research

The system of ALS care must be coordinated with and integrated into the ALS research system. Today, ALS care and research often exist separately, and opportunities are missed to study care delivery and outcomes because the research infrastructure is lacking. The committee envisions the following research role and funding model for the ALS care and research setting in the new network. The concepts are based on the NCI model of centers that provide clinical care and conduct research. There could be clear capabilities and expectations with NINDS core funding at each of the three proposed care and research settings.

Comprehensive ALS Care and Research Centers would lead laboratory, clinical, and population-based research, including biology and genomics, treatment, prevention, behavioral health, health equity, and other social determinants. This would include initiating early-phase clinical trials and leading cooperative clinical trials that include an array of clinical sites, including the regional and community-based clinics, as well as sites outside of the proposed care network to ensure broad patient access to research studies. These comprehensive ALS centers, as coordinating centers, would receive funding from research grants and via foundation- and industry-sponsored research, that it would then distribute to support participating clinical sites, including regional and community-based clinics. This has been a successful approach in several NIH-sponsored multicenter studies.

The Community-Based ALS Care Centers and Regional ALS Centers would be expected to participate in research led by Comprehensive ALS Care and Research Centers, but they could also participate in other research studies, including industry-sponsored studies. Research funding and NINDS designation for the Regional ALS Centers might be modeled after NCI cancer centers, which have the capabilities to lead or participate in federally funded population health research, outcomes research, care delivery research, implementation and dissemination research, and satisfying registry and natural history study enrollment goals. Such funding would also cover personnel support for research navigators to ensure cross-collaboration across care settings in the network.

Connecting VA to the Integrated ALS Care and Research System

As discussed earlier in this chapter, VA is known for strong comprehensive rehabilitative programs for veterans with complex disabilities, much of which were established through congressionally directed funding. The VA ALS system of care follows an interdisciplinary, proactive patient-centric approach, providing early and continued access to specialist consultations, medications, therapies, equipment, and care services, and represents a successful model for non-VA ALS care systems.

Nonetheless, the VA ALS care model does not address several critical issues in the ALS landscape, such as ensuring equitable access to high-quality multidisciplinary ALS care across the country or addressing the projected extreme shortage in the ALS health care and clinical research workforce needed to provide multidisciplinary care and advance therapeutic development (Harp, 2023; Majersik et al., 2021). Moreover, although it does support advanced fellowship training programs in amputation, spinal cord injury, and brain injury, VA does not offer opportunities specific to ALS clinical care. It also does not address the geographic, racial, ethnic, and socioeconomic disparities in access to clinical trials or expanded access programs. While the literature clearly suggests an increased risk of ALS in persons with military service, as concluded in the 2006 Institute of Medicine report *Amyotrophic Lateral Sclerosis in Veterans: Review of the Scientific Literature* (IOM, 2006) no specific work has been undertaken within the U.S. Department of Defense/VA to further understand and propose means to mitigate this increased risk. Furthermore, veterans receiving ALS care within VA clinics have limited access to clinical research, although it does operate a brain bank for postmortem studies of veterans with ALS.

The committee believes that, given the known higher prevalence of ALS in veterans, it is critical to include the VA ALS system of care in the new integrated ALS network of care and research proposed in this report. However, because of rules separating the VA system from other care systems, VA cannot be completely fit into the care and research model proposed earlier in this chapter. Notably, nonveterans are not allowed to receive care at VA clinics, and veterans going outside of the VA system for care will continue to rely on VA for critical benefits, such as DME and medications.

Still, integration would ensure equitable and streamlined access to the highest standard of clinical care for veterans, as well as the ability to participate in clinical trials. With such integration, veterans newly diagnosed with ALS in private care settings would be able to more rapidly connect to comprehensive VA care and resources, and veterans with ALS receiving care in the VA system to access research and additional resources when needed. Clinical trials based at VA facilities would be logistically easier for veterans with ALS to access, removing the barrier of traveling to an outside facility. Finally, given the unique differences in clinical practice between VA ALS clinics and the civilian sector (see Table 4-1), there is ample opportunity for health services research to determine whether these differences improve outcomes for persons with ALS to inform future medical and health policy.

Investment in the VA to achieve these goals would require separate, congressionally mandated funding to build a research infrastructure and organized network of care that would integrate into the proposed model of care under Recommendation 4-1. Without this specific funding source, the VA ALS Centers of Excellence cannot address the gaps outlined earlier in this chapter related to access to clinical research trials and expanded access programs.

Recommendation 4-4: Enhance access to ALS clinical care and research and education opportunities within the U.S. Department of Veterans Affairs (VA).

Congress should allocate specific funding to create a VA network for ALS clinical care, research, education, and innovation to align with the new system of care outlined in this report. VA should use these funds to resolve ALS workforce shortages, ensure access to comprehensive ALS care for veterans regardless of geographic location, increase the number of health professional training opportunities to support ALS care for veterans, and invest in clinical and informatics resources at VA to enhance existing collaboration with the Centers for Disease Control and Prevention ALS registry.

REFERENCES

Ackrivo, J. 2023. Pulmonary care for ALS: Progress, gaps, and paths forward. *Muscle Nerve* 67(5):341–353.

Albanese, A., A. C. Ludolph, C. J. McDermott, P. Corcia, P. van Damme, L. H. van den Berg, O. Hardiman, G. Rinaldi, N. Vanacore, and B. Dickie. 2022. Tauroursodeoxycholic acid in patients with amyotrophic lateral sclerosis: The TUDCA-ALS trial protocol. *Front Neurol* 13:1009113.

Alguire, P. C. 2023. *Understanding capitation.* https://www.acponline.org/about-acp/about-internal-medicine/career-paths/residency-career-counseling/resident-career-counseling-guidance-and-tips/understanding-capitation (accessed April 11, 2024).

ALSA (ALS Association). 2023. ALS around the globe: Improved access to ALS multidisciplinary care—the science of where. In *ALSA Blog.* Arlington, VA.

ALSA. 2024. *thinkALS™ tool.* https://www.als.org/thinkals/thinkals-tool (accessed May 24, 2024).

Andersen, P. M., G. D. Borasio, R. Dengler, O. Hardiman, K. Kollewe, P. N. Leigh, P. F. Pradat, V. Silani, and B. Tomik. 2005. Efns task force on management of amyotrophic lateral sclerosis: Guidelines for diagnosing and clinical care of patients and relatives. *Eur J Neurol* 12(12):921–938.

Arthur, K. C., A. Calvo, T. R. Price, J. T. Geiger, A. Chiò, and B. J. Traynor. 2016. Projected increase in amyotrophic lateral sclerosis from 2015 to 2040. *Nat Commun* 7:12408.

Bedlack, R. S., D. M. Pastula, E. Welsh, D. Pulley, and M. E. Cudkowicz. 2008. Scrutinizing enrollment in ALS clinical trials: Room for improvement? *Amyotroph Lateral Scler* 9(5):257–265.

Belsh, J. M., and P. L. Schiffman. 1996. The amyotrophic lateral sclerosis (ALS) patient perspective on misdiagnosis and its repercussions. *J Neurolog Sci* 139:110–116.

Boylan, K. 2015. Familial amyotrophic lateral sclerosis. *Neurolog Clin* 33(4):807–830.

Boylan, K., T. Levine, C. Lomen-Hoerth, M. Lyon, K. Maginnis, P. Callas, C. Gaspari, and R. Tandan. 2015. Prospective study of cost of care at multidisciplinary ALS centers adhering to American Academy of Neurology (AAN) ALS practice parameters. *Amyotroph Lateral Scler Frontotempor Degener* 17(1–2):119–127.

Carter, C. 2021. *The racial thinking behind ALS diagnosis*. https://www.anthropology-news. org/articles/the-racial-thinking-behind-als-diagnosis/?utm_source=rss&utm_medium=rss &utm_campaign=the-racial-thinking-behind-als-diagnosis#citation (accessed April 11, 2024).

Carter, C. R. 2022. Gaslighting: ALS, anti-Blackness, and medicine. *Fem Anthropol* 3(2): 235–245.

Casey, C. 2023. *Study: Implicit bias, late diagnosis create critical ALS healthcare gap*. https:// news.cuanschutz.edu/news-stories/study-implicit-bias-late-diagnosis-create-critical-als-healthcare-gap (accessed April 11, 2024).

Chen, S., D. Carter, P. Brockenbrough, S. Cox, and K. Gwathmey. 2023. Racial disparities in ALS diagnostic delay: A single center's experience and review of potential contributing factors. *Amyotroph Lateral Scler Frontotempor Degener* 1–7.

Chiò, A., E. Bottacchi, C. Buffa, R. Mutani, and G. Mora. 2006. Positive effects of tertiary centres for amyotrophic lateral sclerosis on outcome and use of hospital facilities. *J Neurol Neurosurg Psychiatry* 77(8):948–950.

Chiò, A., A. Calvo, C. Moglia, L. Mazzini, and G. Mora. 2011. Phenotypic heterogeneity of amyotrophic lateral sclerosis: A population based study. *J Neurol Neurosurg Psychiatry* 82(7):740–746.

Choi, B. C., and A. W. Pak. 2006. Multidisciplinarity, interdisciplinarity and transdisciplinarity in health research, services, education and policy: 1. Definitions, objectives, and evidence of effectiveness. *Clin Invest Med* 29(6):351–364.

Cordesse, V., F. Sidorok, P. Schimmel, J. Holstein, and V. Meininger. 2015. Coordinated care affects hospitalization and prognosis in amyotrophic lateral sclerosis: A cohort study. *BMC Health Services Research* 15(1):134.

Corr, B., E. Frost, B. J. Traynor, and O. Hardiman. 1998. Service provision for patients with ALS/MND: A cost-effective multidisciplinary approach. *J Neurologica Sci* 160:s141–s145.

Cromwell, E. A., J. S. Ostrenga, J. V. Todd, A. Elbert, A. W. Brown, A. Faro, C. H. Goss, and B. C. Marshall. 2023. Cystic fibrosis prevalence in the United States and participation in the Cystic Fibrosis Foundation Patient Registry in 2020. *J Cystic Fibrosis* 22(3):436–442.

de Almeida, F. E. O., A. K. do Carmo Santana, and F. O. de Carvalho. 2021. Multidisciplinary care in amyotrophic lateral sclerosis: A systematic review and meta-analysis. *Neurologic Sci* 42(3):911–923.

Driskell, L. D., M. K. York, P. C. Heyn, M. Sanjak, and C. Macadam. 2019. A guide to understanding the benefits of a multidisciplinary team approach to amyotrophic lateral sclerosis (ALS) treatment. *Arch Phys Med Rehabil* 100(3):583–586.

Fahrner-Scott, K., C. Zapata, D. L. O'Riordan, E. Cohen, L. Rosow, S. Z. Pantilat, C. Lomen-Hoerth, and K. E. Bischoff. 2022. Embedded palliative care for amyotrophic lateral sclerosis: A pilot program and lessons learned. *Neurol Clin Pract* 12(1):68–75.

Falcão de Campos, C., M. Gromicho, H. Uysal, J. Grosskreutz, M. Kuzma-Kozakiewicz, M. Oliveira Santos, S. Pinto, S. Petri, M. Swash, and M. de Carvalho. 2022. Trends in the diagnostic delay and pathway for amyotrophic lateral sclerosis patients across different countries. *Front Neurol* 13:1064619.

Galvin, M., C. Madden, S. Maguire, M. Heverin, A. Vajda, A. Staines, and O. Hardiman. 2015. Patient journey to a specialist amyotrophic lateral sclerosis multidisciplinary clinic: An exploratory study. *BMC Health Serv Res* 15:571.

Galvin, M., P. Ryan, S. Maguire, M. Heverin, C. Madden, A. Vajda, C. Normand, and O. Hardiman. 2017. The path to specialist multidisciplinary care in amyotrophic lateral sclerosis: A population-based study of consultations, interventions and costs. *PLOS One* 12(6):e0179796.

Gelijns, A. C., and S. E. Gabriel. 2012. Looking beyond translation—Integrating clinical research with medical practice. *N Engl J Med* 366(18):1659–1661.

Gladman, M., and L. Zinman. 2015. The economic impact of amyotrophic lateral sclerosis: A systematic review. *Expert Rev Pharmacoecon Outcomes Res* 15(3):439–450.

GlobalData. 2021. *Number of ongoing clinical trials (for drugs) involving amyotrophic lateral sclerosis by phase.* https://www.globaldata.com/data-insights/healthcare/number-of-ongoing-clinical-trials-for-drugs-involving-amyotrophic-lateral-sclerosis-by-phase-503191 (accessed April 11, 2024).

Goyal, N. A., K. Bonar, N. Savic, R. Beau Lejdstrom, J. Wright, J. Mellor, and C. McDermott. 2023. Misdiagnosis of amyotrophic lateral sclerosis in clinical practice in Europe and the U.S.A.: A patient chart review and physician survey. *Amyotroph Lateral Scler Frontotempor Degener* 1–10.

Gwathmey, K., S. Chen, M. Kotay, J. Bingham, S. Patel, J. Prier, D. Carter, P. Brockenbrough, J. Raymond, K. Horton, and P. Mehta. 2023a. *Time to event analysis in Black and White ALS patients: A comparison of the CDC national ALS registry data to that of Virginia Commonwealth University Health ALS Clinic.* Paper presented at 22nd annual meeting of the Northeast ALS Consortium, Clearwater, FL.

Gwathmey, K. G., P. Corcia, C. J. McDermott, A. Genge, S. Sennfält, M. de Carvalho, and C. Ingre. 2023b. Diagnostic delay in amyotrophic lateral sclerosis. *Eur Neurol* 30(9):2595–2601. https://doi.org/10.1111/ene.15874.

Hansen-Flaschen, J. 2021. Respiratory care for patients with amyotrophic lateral sclerosis in the U.S.: In need of support. *JAMA Neurol* 78(9):1047–1048.

Harp, J. J. 2023. The shortage of healthcare workers in the United States: A call to action. *Assessing the need for a comprehensive national health system in the United States.* Advances in healthcare information systems and administration (AHISA) book series, edited by N. Karagiannis, S. R. Goodwin, and D. B. Stewart. Hershey, PA: IGI Global, Information Science Reference. Pp. 123–138.

Haulman, A., A. Geronimo, A. Chahwala, and Z. Simmons. 2020. The use of telehealth to enhance care in ALS and other neuromuscular disorders. *Muscle Nerve* 61(6): 682–691.

HCAA (Home Care Association of America). 2023. *The home care workforce crisis: An industry report and call to action.* Washington, DC: Home Care Association of America.

Helleman, J., E. T. Kruitwagen, L. H. van den Berg, J. M. A. Visser-Meily, and A. Beelen. 2020. The current use of telehealth in ALS care and the barriers to and facilitators of implementation: A systematic review. *Amyotroph Lateral Scler Frontotempor Degener* 21(3–4):167–182.

Hill, L., N. Ndugga, and S. Artiga. 2023. *Key data on health and health care by race and ethnicity.* San Francisco, CA: Kaiser Family Foundation.

Hogden, A., and A. Crook. 2017. Patient-centered decision making in amyotrophic lateral sclerosis: Where are we? *Neurodegener Dis Manag* 7(6):377–386.

Horton, D. K., S. Graham, R. Punjani, G. Wilt, W. Kaye, K. Maginnis, L. Webb, J. Richman, R. Bedlack, E. Tessaro, and P. Mehta. 2018. A spatial analysis of amyotrophic lateral sclerosis (ALS) cases in the United States and their proximity to multidisciplinary ALS clinics, 2013. *Amyotroph Lateral Scler Frontotempor Degener* 19(1–2):126–133.

I AM ALS. 2024. *ALS clinic map.* https://www.iamals.org/get-help/find-your-als-clinic (accessed March 21, 2024).

IOM (Institute of Medicine). 2006. *Amyotrophic lateral sclerosis in veterans: Review of the scientific literature.* Washington, DC: The National Academies Press.

Ipsos. 2019. *Clinical trials survey.* Washington, DC: I AM ALS.

Katyal, N., and R. Govindarajan. 2017. Shortcomings in the current amyotrophic lateral sclerosis trials and potential solutions for improvement. *Front Neurol* 8:521.

Knapp, E. A., A. K. Fink, C. H. Goss, A. Sewall, J. Ostrenga, C. Dowd, A. Elbert, K. M. Petren, and B. C. Marshall. 2016. The Cystic Fibrosis Foundation Patient Registry. Design and methods of a national observational disease registry. *Ann Am Thorac Soc* 13(7):1173–1179.

Koroshetz, W. J. 2023. *A path forward: Strategic priorities for amyotrophic lateral sclerosis (ALS).* https://www.ninds.nih.gov/news-events/directors-messages/all-directors-messages/path-forward-strategic-priorities-amyotrophic-lateral-sclerosis-als (accessed April 11, 2024).

Majersik, J. J., A. Ahmed, I. A. Chen, H. Shill, G. P. Hanes, V. S. Pelak, J. L. Hopp, A. Omuro, B. Kluger, and T. Leslie-Mazwi. 2021. A shortage of neurologists—we must act now: A report from the AAN 2019 Transforming Leaders Program. *Neurol* 96(24):1122–1134.

Market.US. 2023. *Global amyotrophic lateral sclerosis treatment market.* New York: Market.US.

Matharan, M., S. Mathis, S. Bonabaud, L. Carla, A. Soulages, and G. Le Masson. 2020. Minimizing the diagnostic delay in amyotrophic lateral sclerosis: The role of nonneurologist practitioners. *Neurol Res Int* 2020:1473981.

McDonald, C. M., and W. M. Fowler, Jr. 2012. The role of the neuromuscular medicine and physiatry specialists in the multidisciplinary management of neuromuscular disease. *Phys Med Rehabil Clin N Am* 23(3):475–493.

MDA (Muscular Dystrophy Association). 2023. *MDA care centers: A national network of expert care.* https://mdaquest.org/mda-care-centers-a-national-network-of-expert-care (accessed April 11, 2024).

Mehta, P., J. Raymond, M. K. Han, T. Larson, J. D. Berry, S. Paganoni, H. Mitsumoto, R. S. Bedlack, and D. K. Horton. 2021. Recruitment of patients with amyotrophic lateral sclerosis for clinical trials and epidemiological studies: Descriptive study of the National ALS Registry's research notification mechanism. *J Med Internet Res* 23(12):e28021.

Mehta, P., J. Raymond, Y. Zhang, R. Punjani, M. Han, T. Larson, O. Muravov, R. H. Lyles, and D. K. Horton. 2023. Prevalence of amyotrophic lateral sclerosis in the United States, 2018. *Amyotroph Lateral Scler Frontotempor Degener* 24(7–8):702–708.

Metzl, J. M., and H. Hansen. 2014. Structural competency: Theorizing a new medical engagement with stigma and inequality. *Soc Sci Med* 103:126–133.

Miller, C., S. Apple, J. S. Paige, T. Grabowsky, O. Shukla, W. Agnese, and C. Merrill. 2021. Current and future projections of amyotrophic lateral sclerosis in the United States using administrative claims data. *Neuroepidemiol* 55(4):275–285.

Miller, R. G., C. E. Jackson, E. J. Kasarskis, J. D. England, D. Forshew, W. Johnston, S. Kalra, J. S. Katz, H. Mitsumoto, J. Rosenfeld, C. Shoesmith, M. J. Strong, and S. C. Woolley. 2009. Practice parameter update: The care of the patient with amyotrophic lateral sclerosis: Multidisciplinary care, symptom management, and cognitive/behavioral impairment (an evidence-based review). Report of the Quality Standards Subcommittee of the American Academy of Neurology. *Neurology* 73(15):1227–1233.

Mintzi, M. 2022. *Care model case study: Patient and family-centered specialty care medical home.* Minneapolis, MN: American Academy of Neurology.

Mitchell, J. D., P. Callagher, J. Gardham, C. Mitchell, M. Dixon, R. Addison-Jones, W. Bennett, and M. R. O'Brien. 2010. Timelines in the diagnostic evaluation of people with suspected amyotrophic lateral sclerosis (ALS)/motor neuron disease (MND)—a 20-year review: Can we do better? *Amyotroph Lateral Scler* 11(6):537–541.

Morren, J. A., C. Rheaume, and E. P. Pioro. 2023. Self-reported factors contributing to delay in ALS diagnosis among primary care providers in a large Ohio-based US healthcare network. *J Neurol Sci* 445:120532.

Obermann, M., and M. Lyon. 2015. Financial cost of amyotrophic lateral sclerosis: A case study. *Amyotroph Lateral Scler Frontotempor Degener* 16(1–2):54–57.

Paganoni, S., K. Nicholson, F. Leigh, K. Swoboda, D. Chad, K. Drake, K. Haley, M. Cudkowicz, and J. D. Berry. 2017. Developing multidisciplinary clinics for neuromuscular care and research. *Muscle Nerve* 56(5):848–858.

Paganoni, S., S. Hendrix, S. P. Dickson, N. Knowlton, E. A. Macklin, J. D. Berry, M. A. Elliott, et al. 2021. Long-term survival of participants in the CENTAUR trial of sodium phenylbutyrate-taurursodiol in amyotrophic lateral sclerosis. *Muscle Nerve* 63(1):31–39.

Palese, F., A. Sartori, G. Logroscino, and F. E. Pisa. 2019. Predictors of diagnostic delay in amyotrophic lateral sclerosis: A cohort study based on administrative and electronic medical records data. *Amyotroph Lateral Scler Frontotempor Degener* 20(3–4):176–185.

Raymond, J., B. Oskarsson, P. Mehta, and K. Horton. 2019. Clinical characteristics of a large cohort of US participants enrolled in the National Amyotrophic Lateral Sclerosis (ALS) Registry, 2010–2015. *Amyotroph Lateral Scler Frontotempor Degener* 20(5–6):413–420.

Richards, D., J. A. Morren, and E. P. Pioro. 2021. Time to diagnosis and factors affecting diagnostic delay in amyotrophic lateral sclerosis. *Amyotrophic Lateral Sclerosis*, edited by T. Araki. Brisbane, Australia: Exon Publications.

Schellenberg, K. L., and G. Hansen. 2018. Patient perspectives on transitioning to amyotrophic lateral sclerosis multidisciplinary clinics. *J Multidisciplin Healthcare* 11:519–524.

Skulstad Johanson, G. A., O. B. Tysnes, and T. L. Bjerknes. 2022. Use of off-label drugs and nutrition supplements among patients with amyotrophic lateral sclerosis in Norway. *Neurol Res Int* 1789946.

Stephens, H. E., J. Young, S. H. Felgoise, and Z. Simmons. 2015. A qualitative study of multidisciplinary ALS clinic use in the United States. *Amyotroph Lateral Scler Frontotemporal Degener* 17(1–2):55–61.

Thakore, N. J., B. R. Lapin, E. P. Pioro, and L. S. Aboussouan. 2019. Variation in noninvasive ventilation use in amyotrophic lateral sclerosis. *Neurol* 93(3):e306–e316.

Traynor, B. J., M. Alexander, B. Corr, E. Frost, and O. Hardiman. 2003. Effect of a multidisciplinary amyotrophic lateral sclerosis (ALS) clinic on ALS survival: A population based study, 1996–2000. *J Neurol Neurosurg Psychiatry* 74(9):1258–1261.

Valor Healthcare. n.d. *What percentage of ALS patients are veterans?* https://valorhealthcare.com/what-percentage-of-als-patients-are-veterans (accessed April 11, 2024).

VHA (Veterans Health Administration). 2021. *Amyotrophic lateral sclerosis system of care.* Washington, DC: Veterans Health Administration.

Woodcock, J., R. Araojo, T. Thompson, and G. A. Puckrein. 2021. Integrating research into community practice—Toward increased diversity in clinical trials. *N Engl J Med* 385(15):1351–1353.

5

Advancing ALS Research and Accelerating Therapeutic Development

ABSTRACT

This chapter considers the many areas of research necessary to advance our understanding of amyotrophic lateral sclerosis (ALS) and measure progress toward making it a more livable disease. It first considers the drug development ecosystem, identifies major challenges to developing and testing drug candidates, and makes the case for establishing a clinical trials network to accelerate the development of new therapies, both pharmacologic and supportive. The chapter highlights the need for disease biomarkers to enable earlier detection of ALS, increase recruitment for clinical trials, and assess therapeutic efficacy in clinical trials and the importance of identifying new targets for developing new drug and gene therapies. It also discusses the use of patient registries in informing care and research for various diseases and the importance of bolstering the capabilities of the existing National ALS Registry. The chapter discusses ways to expand the National ALS Registry and integrate it into a comprehensive data platform featuring other sources of data. The chapter then discusses nonpharmacological therapies that can help relieve and manage disease symptoms and make ALS a more livable disease and notes the need for studies to identify which therapies and combinations of therapies work best to prolong the duration and quality of life and to improve the quality of interventions involving these therapies.

Immediately preceding and during the time this study committee was working, the U.S. Food and Drug Administration (FDA) approved two

135

new ALS drugs (AMX0035/Relyvrio and tofersen/Qalsody). However, in March 2024, while the committee was finishing its work on this report, the company developing AMX0035/Relyvrio, announced the latest results of a Phase 3 trial in which the drug performed no better than placebo. In April 2024, the company that developed Relyvrio announced the drug would be removed from the market in the United States and Canada. It is not within the statement of task for this study to suggest regulatory approval or disapproval of any specific new ALS drug applications FDA will consider. However, the committee saw a unique opportunity in the therapeutic development space to provide broader recommended actions for industry, ALS nonprofit organizations, public–private partnerships, researchers, and regulators to make use of the research and clinical trials network discussed in Chapter 4 to foster a more detailed understanding of the root causes of ALS, how they manifest themselves as disease symptoms, and how to use that new knowledge to accelerate the development of new therapies that can improve the lived experiences of individuals with ALS.

ALS DRUG DEVELOPMENT THROUGH THE YEARS

The history of drug development for ALS is filled with many failures and too few successful drugs. Even the four drugs (Qalsody/tofersen, Radicava/edaravone, Rilutek/riluzole, and Nuedexta) and two additional formulations of riluzole (Tiglutik/thickened riluzole and Exservan/riluzole oral film) FDA has approved for ALS are based on limited clinical benefit or likelihood of clinical benefit. And one ALS drug (Relyvrio) was being removed from the market as of April 2024 due to lack of clinical benefit. Over the past decade, numerous research advances have identified a wide range of potential therapeutic pathways and potential drug targets and genes associated with the disease. However, the heterogeneity and complex biological pathways of ALS have slowed the development of biomarker research. Diagnostic delay and inadequate eligibility criteria affect the ability of study populations to appropriately reflect the heterogeneity of ALS (Katyal and Govindarajan, 2017). In many disease spaces, gene variants associated with the disease have indicated potential targets for drug and biomarker development. However, both sporadic ALS and familial ALS are associated with mutations in at least one of more than 50 disease causative genes and 120 genetic variants that increase the risk or modify the ALS phenotype (Fang et al., 2022). Each of these could point to a therapeutic target, and many are being studied (Mead et al., 2023).

A 2023 review of ALS clinical trials identified more than 60 compounds with a variety of mechanisms of action targeting different biochemical and genetic processes that researchers have evaluated as potential treatments for ALS (Mead et al., 2023). Figure 5-1 show the major ALS pathophysiological targets currently being pursued.

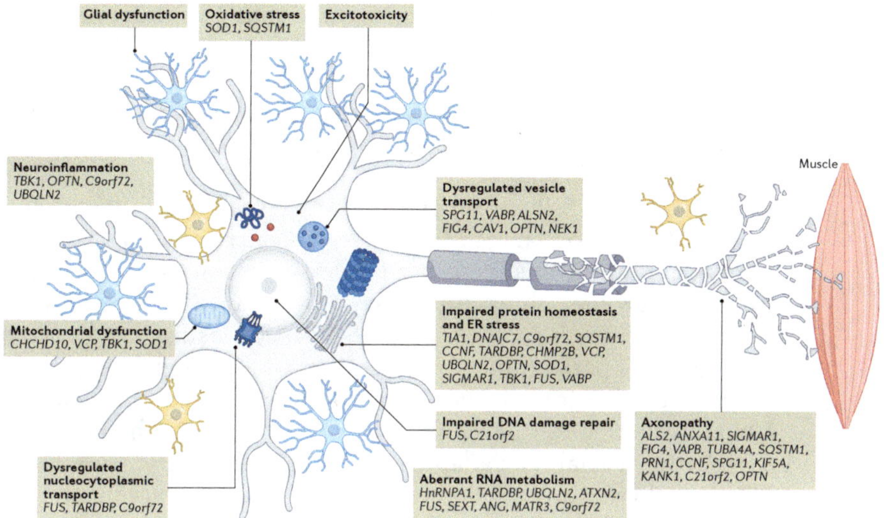

FIGURE 5-1 ALS pathophysiology, genetic causes, and risk factors.
SOURCE: Mead et al., 2023.

ALS CLINICAL TRIALS AND NATURAL HISTORY STUDIES

Since 1995, FDA has approved five drugs and two additional formulations of one of those drugs for treating ALS. In addition to these medications, several other candidates are in clinical trials. One estimate is that 53 drug development programs that include a focus on ALS were underway in 2022 (Mead et al., 2023). Industry, academia, the federal government, and nonprofit organizations are all involved in some manner in efforts to develop therapeutics for ALS, often in collaboration across sectors. Examples include:

- The Network for Excellence in Neuroscience Clinical Trials (NeuroNEXT) is funded by the National Institute of Neurological Disorders and Stroke (NINDS) and is designed to increase efficiency of clinical trials, expand the capability of NINDS to test promising new therapies, and respond quickly as opportunities arise to test promising new treatments for people with neurological disorders. NeuroNEXT has more than 10 clinical trial sites in the United States (NeuroNEXT, 2024).
- Northeast ALS Consortium (NEALS), founded in 1995, includes 156 trial-ready sites for ALS. NEALS has successfully partnered with industry and academic researchers to conduct nearly 80 high-quality ALS studies for more than 25 years. NEALS

provides all sites with comprehensive training in outcome measures and site management so NEALS can quickly initiate new trials and produce high-quality data. NEALS has also established a repository of serum, plasma, cerebrospinal fluid, whole blood, extracted DNA, and urine samples from NEALS research studies (NEALS, 2024).

- The HEALEY ALS Platform Trial,[1] led by researchers at the Healey & AMG Center for ALS at Massachusetts General Hospital (MGH), is a collaboration involving the Healey Center for ALS; NEALS; Barrow Neurological Institute; Berry Consultants; 78 participating U.S. sites overseen by one, central, SMART-institutional review board;[2] ALS patient members serving on steering committees; several pharmaceutical and biotech industry collaborators; and numerous biomarker development research groups. The HEALEY ALS Platform Trial is an adaptive clinical trial that serves as a Phase 2/3 clinical efficacy trial that in its first 3 years has accepted eight experimental drug regimens for testing.[3]

- The ALS Therapy Development Institute (TDI) is a nonprofit biotechnology company that conducts preclinical, clinical, and translational research and has screened more than 400 potential treatments for ALS in preclinical models. As part of its efforts, ALS TDI established the ALS Research Collaborative (ARC) to collect natural history data from people with ALS and merge those data with genomics, proteomics, and metabolomics data to empower the larger research community through the ARC Data Commons.[4] ALS TDI has also developed a potential therapeutic that in May 2022 successfully completed a Phase 2a clinical trial (ALS TDI, 2022).

In addition to networks that conduct clinical trials, other consortia generate data to inform the design of clinical trials and accelerate progress on finding potential therapeutics that would enter clinical trials. Examples include:

- The Access for All in ALS Clinical Research Consortium (ALL ALS) funded by NINDS in 2023 will provide a large scalable clinical research infrastructure and has the goal of facilitating research

---

[1]Platform trials enable testing multiple drug candidates and biomarkers in the same trial against a common control or usual care group according to predefined rules. They are open ended in that new candidates can be added, assessed, and removed as the trial progresses.

[2]Additional information is available at https://smartirb.org (accessed May 10, 2024).

[3]Adaptive clinical trials are designed to study multiple targeted therapies to a single disease in a perpetual manner, with therapies allowed to enter or leave the platform on the basis of a predefined decision algorithm (Adaptive Clinical Trials Coalition, 2019; Quintana et al., 2023).

[4]Available at https://www.als.net/arc/data-commons (accessed May 10, 2024).

aimed at obtaining mechanistic insights into ALS heterogeneity and identifying therapeutic targets and biomarkers (see Chapter 1 for additional information).

- In September 2022, FDA and the National Institutes of Health (NIH) established the Critical Path for Rare Neurodegenerative Diseases (CP-RND), a public–private partnership that the Critical Path Institute (C-Path) will lead. This effort will involve members of ALS patient communities, pharmaceutical and biotechnology companies, regulators, and ALS advocacy organizations, who will work together to set the initiative's priorities for patient-focused drug development (C-Path, 2024). (See Chapter 1 for additional information.)

- The Pooled Resource Open-Access ALS Clinical Trials Database (PRO-ACT) is a data platform, created in partnership with NEALS, that houses the largest collection of ALS clinical trials datasets. PRO-ACT contains placebo data from 11,675 people with ALS who participated in clinical trials sponsored by industry, foundations, and academia (NCRI, 2024)

- AnswerALS enrolled 1,000 participants from eight sites across the nation who provided biospecimens that the AnswerALS research team used to generate induced pluripotent brain stem cells from each participant. Every sample went through genomic, proteomic, and transcriptomic analysis to produce a personalized data of ALS-specific information. In collaboration with experts in machine learning and big data informatics, this biological data will be mined to uncover ALS causes, subtypes, pathways gone awry, and drug targets. These data will serve as the foundation for new clinical trials, suggest new ways to subgroup patients to better discover successful drugs, and identify drug-responsive biomarkers or diagnostics (Answer ALS, 2024).

- The European Network to Cure ALS (ENCALS) is a network of European ALS centers with aims including the development of a European ALS research network with database and biobank, collaboration between funding agencies to sponsor investigator-initiated research projects, reaching consensus on a classification of ALS suitable for European research projects, and studying novel designs for the assessment of efficacy of new therapies for ALS (ENCALS, 2024).

- The Treatment Research Initiative to Cure ALS (TRICALS), another European research consortium, includes 48 research centers in 16 countries, people with ALS, and ALS foundations that collaborate with pharmaceutical and biotechnology companies. This consortium focuses on using data to identify and develop biomarkers for different types of ALS, improving the design of clinical trials, and establishing an international registry of individuals with ALS to enable easy access to clinical trials (TRICALS, 2024).

Each ALS research initiative or network is uniquely structured and funded to meet its mission. The committee considered some of the attributes of three ALS research networks and resources currently in operation or under development in the United States today (see Table 5-1) to better understand the gaps and opportunities in the ALS research ecosystem.

TABLE 5-1 Attributes of Three ALS Research Networks and Resources

	Network for Excellence in Neuroscience Clinical Trials (NeuroNEXT)	Northeast ALS (NEALS) Consortium	Access for All in ALS (ALL ALS)
Origin and scope of work	Funded by NINDS since 2011. Exploratory Phase 2 trials only. Network for many diseases, including ALS.	Established in 1995 as an academic research consortium. All clinical trials (Phase 1, 2 and 3), natural history, and observational studies supported.	Established via NINDS awards in October 2023. Natural history study focused.
Funding model	NINDS funded. Coordination centers; infrastructural support for sites for supporting hiring, training and salary for research coordinator(s), nurse(s), and principal investigator's time. Subject to annual progress and productivity metrics for renewal.	Original donors include ALS Association's TREAT ALS Network, Muscular Dystrophy Association, and others. No federal funding. A voluntary network of ad hoc sites that contract with affiliated sponsors. Funded mainly by per participant fee for projects.	NINDS funded. Coordination center operational costs; infrastructural support includes a dedicated navigator for recruitment and retention activities.
Size and output	More than 10 academic sites in United States; no ALS trials to date.	More than 155 sites in United States and internationally. 18 ALS trials in 2023 (8 completed, 10 ongoing).	34 sites in the United States and Puerto Rico being launched in 2024.

TABLE 5-1 Continued

	Network for Excellence in Neuroscience Clinical Trials (NeuroNEXT)	Northeast ALS (NEALS) Consortium	Access for All in ALS (ALL ALS)
Operations and infrastructure	Central infrastructure funded through NINDS. MGH NCRI as clinical coordinating center. University of Iowa as data coordinating center. Smart IRB and Central reliance agreements for all sites.	Industry or other trial sponsors contract with MGH NCRI as an ARO or use commercial CRO for trial operations. No reliance agreements for sites (all member sites receive standardized trial outcomes training, educational support and research updates, recruitment and retention support). Central IRB selection per sponsor's choice.	Central infrastructure funded through NINDS. MGH serves as central IRB.
Scientific Advisory Board	Vets drugs for entering the network; makes go/no go decisions on whether a drug is scientifically valid for clinical trials.	Provides design and development input to industry investigators but does not make go/no go decisions.	No interventional drugs tested. Oversight of the research consortium provided by NIH and FNIH via AMP ALS.
Data and safety oversight	Data safety monitoring board approved by NINDS.	Ad hoc assembled by sponsor outside of network.	Observational study monitoring board approved by NINDS.
Data repository and sharing	NIH specified central data and sample repositories; mandated sharing.	No data-sharing requirements for trial sponsors using NEALS. Sponsors have the option to share placebo data in a centralized database but not required.	NIH specified central data and sample repositories; mandated sharing.

NOTE: AMP ALS = Accelerated Medicines Partnership for ALS; ARO = academic research organization; CRO = contract research organization; FNIH = Foundation for the National Institutes of Health; IRB = institutional review board; MGH = Massachusetts General Hospital; NCRI = Neurological Clinical Research Institute; NIH = National Institutes of Health; NINDS = National Institute of Neurological Disorders and Stroke.
SOURCES: NEALS, 2024; NeuroNEXT, 2024; NIH, 2023.

Although each of these networks provides a useful resource, the differences among them make it difficult to integrate results across them and to maximize each trial's possibilities. Today, many industry-sponsored ALS trials are run out of NEALS which provides access to many sites and significant flexibility to the sponsor in deciding which therapeutic candidates to test and whether data will be shared once the trial is complete. NEALS can provide a large network of trial-ready sites and clinicians, community engagement and education and standardized clinical outcomes training, but it does not have the scalable trial infrastructure, harmonized data banks, and funding model that an expanded, supported, NIH network could offer. Also, the development of the ALS clinical trials workforce is hampered under the currently fragmented research networks. The committee believes a centralized ALS clinical trials network led by NIH would provide the best of each current network and harmonize approaches and support to see improvements in ALS trial success. Similarly structured cancer clinical trials networks, such as the National Cancer Institute's National Clinical Trials Network, have shown to be high impact for the field and benefited from NIH leadership. The committee suggests that the following areas would be improved under an NIH-led ALS clinical trials network:

- Data sharing—currently not required for studies run outside of NIH. A centralized data sharing requirement, with accountability, would advance open science for ALS.
- Infrastructure—currently variable, requiring research teams to be assembled anew for each research study. Sustained research teams and tools would be better prepared to launch and run trials effectively.
- Equity—clinical trial opportunities are currently inequitably allocated across the ALS population and focused on large academic centers. A centralized clinical trial network would be designed to bring in new, rural sites and adopt remote monitoring to improve the clinical trial experience for more people with ALS.
- Community engagement—trainings, educational opportunities, and partnerships among persons with ALS lived experience and ALS researchers are critical to the success of drug development efforts. Centralized supports and best practices for these activities are needed so they can take place in greater numbers across the country.
- Governance—variable across networks today but a centralized network could apply a coherent approach to selecting compounds to be tested in the network and involve steering committees that include people with ALS lived experience.
- Innovation—complexity in ALS clinical trial and specialized expertise often required. Innovations that improve the experience for people with ALS and speed the testing of new therapies deserve widespread consideration and adoption.

ALS Natural History Studies

Unlike clinical trials, natural history or observational studies are not meant to produce interventions to try to change outcomes such as disease progression or survival. Natural history studies involve following a group of people living with ALS over time to see how their disease progresses; these studies can collect biospecimens and clinical data to investigate genetic causes of ALS, identify potential biomarkers, and explore the role of environmental factors in ALS development. Cohort-based natural history studies focus on a specific group of people with a common characteristic, such as individuals in the military.

Data from natural history studies can serve as concurrent controls, and in some cases replace the internal controls used in randomized, placebo-controlled clinical trials. Opportunities to reduce the burden of clinical trial participation are important for diseases such as ALS with high and predictable mortality or progressive morbidity when it may not always be feasible to have individuals on a control arm (Jahanshahi et al., 2021). A robust, perpetually ongoing natural history study with a diverse, nationwide sample could reduce the need for placebo controls (Ghadessi et al., 2020). However, using natural history studies as external controls can be limited in their usefulness for heterogenous disease such as ALS and requires case-by-case assessment. As FDA notes, historical controls can be effective if the natural history of the disease is well defined which is not the case yet for ALS (FDA, 2023)

Should the natural history of ALS become better understood, using natural history studies to serve as an external control could become increasingly important as investigators bring more gene-targeted ALS drugs to human clinical trials. Drug development in oncology has extensively used natural history studies as concurrent controls (Collignon et al., 2021; Mishra-Kalyani et al., 2022).

Examples of natural history studies include:

- The CP-RND operated under C-Path will focus on increasing understanding of disease pathogenesis and natural history by quantifying disease progression. The model uses a pre-competitive framework to allow commercial developers to bring data and shared learnings to the table and engage with regulators, patient communities, and advocacy organizations (C-Path, 2024).
- The ALS/Motor Neuron Disease (MND) Natural History Consortium operates under the Center for Innovation & Bioinformatics of the NCRI at MGH and collects real-world data about ALS to inform research and clinical trial design. The consortium includes academic medical centers in the United States and Europe and is a multidisciplinary, clinic-based registry that is prospectively

and longitudinally capturing clinical information about the disease process from people living with ALS. All patients with a diagnosis of ALS or other motor neuron diseases are eligible to be enrolled during a routine multidisciplinary clinic visit (Berger et al., 2023; CIB, 2024).

- REFINE ALS is a fully enrolled biomarker study launched after FDA approved Radicava and is led by a collaboration between MGH and Mitsubishi Tanabe Pharma America. In this study, the collaborators are following 300-plus individuals with ALS for clinical and biofluid biomarker trends following initiation of Radicava treatment. This study aims to better understand the effects of this medication on disease progression and provide insights into its mechanism of action and biomarker trends.

- The ALS Research Collaborative Natural History Study, operated by ALS TDI, is the longest running natural history study in ALS. Participants share data on their movement, lifestyle, medical history, genetics, biomarkers, voice recordings, and patient cell biology to inform ALS research (ALS TDI, 2024).

- Target ALS Biofluid Consortium, comprising 10 ALS clinics from around the world, launched a natural history study in 2021 to generate the most comprehensive collection of longitudinal biofluid samples and data from at least 800 ALS and 200 healthy control cases. The study is collecting detailed clinical and demographic information, speech and respiratory functional data, multi-omic datasets, and longitudinal biofluid collection of cerebrospinal fluid, blood, and urine.

Although a variety of mechanisms exist for conducting clinical trials and natural history studies, a centralized, dedicated ALS clinical trials network that builds on and brings together existing ALS clinical trial consortia could provide a coherent approach to clinical trials and natural history studies that permits faster answers to multiple questions at once. A clinical trials network would need to include representatives of the entire pool of individuals living with ALS, particularly individuals representing diverse ethnic and racial populations, and it would need to be strategic in site selection to expand the opportunities for individuals to participate who might otherwise not be able to or want to travel a long distance to participate in a clinical trial. To be most effective, the clinical trials network would need to be coordinated for operations, outcomes, quality trainings, and oversight within the integrated ALS clinical care and research network the committee proposes in Chapter 4.

An expanded and coordinated ALS clinical trials network could facilitate a larger array of human studies, such as first-in-human clinical trials, personalized gene therapy trials for ultrarare forms of ALS, and large Phase 3 trials. It could also provide access to clinical trials for a larger and more diverse population of individuals with ALS. Such a clinical trial network can be modeled after and built on already existing successful models such as NeuroNext and NEALS. These two clinical trial networks could serve as a base from which to build a larger, more diverse ALS-specific network.

Such a clinical trials network dedicated to ALS would create an exciting opportunity for scores of multidisciplinary ALS centers in diverse geographic areas to bring clinical trial and biomarker research closer to ALS individuals' homes across the nation, which otherwise would not be possible.

Recommendation 5-1: Create an ALS clinical trials network.

The National Institute of Neurological Disorders and Stroke should ensure the existence of a dedicated ALS clinical trials network distributed across diverse geographic regions in the United States, coordinated and funded by the National Institutes of Health. To be most effective, the ALS clinical trials network should be integrated with the hub-and-spoke clinical care network recommended in this report.

DEVELOPING ALS BIOMARKERS AND OTHER CLINICAL ENDPOINTS TO SERVE AS INDICATORS OF DRUG EFFICACY

One challenge for drug development, recruitment for clinical trials, and disease diagnosis is the heterogeneity of ALS in terms of how and when symptoms develop, how quickly it progresses, its resemblance to other motor neuron and neurological diseases, and in the genes and proteins associated with developing ALS. For the most part, ALS is diagnosed based on the appearance of certain clinical features, which both slows the diagnostic process and can confound drug development and stratifying people with ALS for participating in clinical trials. To address this problem, researchers are searching for biomarkers—specific molecular, biochemical, genetic, and imaging characteristics that can serve as a more accurate indicator of early disease confirmation, track disease progression, and detect biological treatment responses in trials using surrogate biomarkers before clinical benefits appear (see Box 5-1). Blood tests and magnetic resonance imaging, for example, are common biomarkers for a variety of diseases.

TDP-43, a protein that regulates how RNA is processed, is one focus of recent research efforts because TDP-43 dysfunction is linked to almost all individuals with ALS and about half of those with frontotemporal dementia (FTD) (NINDS, 2024). Recent research further advanced our understanding of how cryptic exons could be involved in the disease

---

BOX 5-1
Types of Biomarkers

The U.S. Food and Drug Administration (FDA) and the National Institutes of Health (NIH) developed the following definitions for different types of biomarkers, each with its own use in clinical research and treatment.

- *Diagnostic biomarkers* detect or confirm the presence of a disease or condition of interest or identify an individual with a subtype of the disease. Such biomarkers may be used to identify people with a disease and redefine the classification of the disease.
- *Monitoring biomarkers* can be measured serially to assess the status of a disease or medical condition for evidence of exposure to a medical product or environmental agent, or to detect an effect of a medical product or biological agent. Monitoring is a broad concept, so there is overlap with other categories of biomarkers as described below.
- *Pharmacodynamic/response biomarkers* are those whose levels change in response to exposure to a medical product or an environmental agent.
- *Predictive biomarkers* are defined by the finding that the presence or change in the biomarker predicts an individual or group of individuals are more likely to experience a favorable or unfavorable effect from the exposure to a medical product or environmental agent.
- *Prognostic biomarkers* identify the likelihood of a clinical event, disease recurrence, or disease progression in patients with a disease or medical condition of interest. Prognostic biomarkers are associated with differential disease outcomes, but predictive biomarkers discriminate those who will respond or not respond to therapy.
- *Safety biomarkers* are measured before and after an exposure to a medical intervention or environmental agent to indicate the likelihood, presence, or extent of a toxicity as an adverse event.
- *Susceptibility/risk biomarkers* indicate the potential for developing a disease or medical condition.
- *Surrogate biomarkers* are correlated with and explain the change in clinical outcome.

SOURCE: FDA-NIH Biomarker Working Group, 2016.

---

process and how diseases involving TDP-43 dysfunction could be identified before symptoms appear by testing an individual's cerebrospinal fluid (NINDS, 2024; Seddighi et al., 2024).

Having clinically proven, easy-to-measure screening and diagnostic biomarkers that can confirm ALS at the earliest stages of disease onset can accelerate early recognition of the disease, diagnosis, and initiation of therapies and approved medications. As Chapter 2 notes, diagnosing ALS in its earliest manifestation would enable more individuals to meet inclusion criteria for participating in clinical trials. Validated diagnostic biomarkers would address diagnostic uncertainties, reduce the number of referrals to nonspecialists, and eliminate potential confounding factors that can produce misleading clinical trial results. For example, if a potential therapeutic agent targets a specific genetic mutation, the odds of a clinical trial achieving statistically significant results would increase if the patient population being studied was restricted to individuals with that specific mutation, rather than being open to anyone with ALS.

Ideally, one biomarker or a combination of several biomarkers would provide presymptomatic diagnosis of ALS, which would be valuable for individuals with a family history of ALS and could enable developing and using therapies that stop or even reverse the disease process before it damages too many nerve cells. Currently, FDA accepts slowing of disease-related decline, stabilization, and improvement of function in daily activities, as measured using either the Revised Amyotrophic Lateral Sclerosis Functional Rating Scale (ALSFRS-R)[5] or a scale of combined function and survival outcomes (Berry et al., 2013; Cedarbaum et al., 1999; Quintana et al., 2023), as a clinical trial endpoint indicative of drug efficacy (FDA, 2019).

TRADE-OFFS IN ALS DRUG DEVELOPMENT AND APPROVAL

As of December 2023, FDA had approved several drugs to treat ALS or its symptoms. Several of these approvals have not been without controversy, stemming in part from a belief that some drugs might have been approved too soon, without sufficient data on efficacy because of pressure from advocates and people with ALS regarding the urgent need for new medications and the desire to have anything to help people living with ALS with this devastating and fatal disease. Considering the appropriate balance between achieving confidence in an ALS drug's benefits and accessing the drug as quickly as possible is a complex and often emotionally charged issue. Approving drugs despite considerable residual uncertainty

---

[5] ALSFRS-R is a validated instrument for monitoring the progression of disability in patients with ALS by measuring 12 aspects of physical function, ranging from one's ability to swallow and use utensils to climbing stairs and breathing (Cedarbaum et al., 1999).

complicates clinical decision making, as people with ALS and their physicians must weigh adverse effects and other burdens against uncertain benefits. Without compelling efficacy data, it will not be clear which patients should be prescribed which drugs, or how they should be used alone or in combination to maximize benefit. In addition, adverse effects such as nausea, diarrhea, or dry skin may sound minor compared to the risks associated with a fatal disease, but adverse effects that may be tolerable for a drug that works are intolerable for a drug that does not. When there is inadequate evidence of benefit, expanded access programs offer a mechanism for ineligible for clinical trials to receive treatment while definitive data are being collected.

Even after FDA approval, access to new drugs is uneven for persons living with ALS today. Not everyone living with ALS will receive new drugs. Reasons for this include:

- Their insurance company will not pay for the drug given unclear efficacy.
- The person with ALS who wants to take the drug does not satisfy the criteria set in clinical trials to support the drug.
- The drug is prohibitively expensive with or without insurance coverage.
- The drug is administered in a manner that is impossible or unappealing for the person living with ALS.
- The clinic or care setting for a person living with ALS cannot support administration of the drug or the process of requesting insurance approval.
- The person with ALS may be among the estimated half of persons living with ALS today not receiving care in a multidisciplinary setting and therefore are unconnected to the latest ALS interventions.

Throughout the phases of developing, approving, and accessing a new ALS drug there are many considerations and trade-offs that deserve attention and discussion among a wide range of individuals affected by ALS. The committee encourages ALS organizations to host conversations about these trade-offs and include nonprofit advocacy organizations, academic research groups, and regulators. Participants could include persons living with ALS; families affected by ALS in the past, present, or likely future; at-risk genetic carriers; ALS clinicians; drug developers; and others. The goals of these conversations could include learning about and discussing the trade-offs arising between the urgent need for effective therapeutic interventions; the importance of strong evidence of clinical benefit and safety; and the implications for FDA approval, patient autonomy, payer coverage, and future development of ALS drugs. The committee offers these ideas for launching these discussions on trade-offs in the drug development and approval process:

- NIH and NINDS could support research to further understand and address these trade-offs as they arise, specifically in the context of ALS, and to improve the use of the expanded access pathway to ease the tension in demanding earlier drug approvals.
- FDA could seek comment on these trade-offs to better understand and appreciate the diversity of views on their implications in the ALS community. Such input might help FDA with difficult decisions on what counts as clinically meaningful benefit and adequate evidence in making critical approval decisions.
- ALS organizations could offer educational resources and create opportunities for people living with ALS and their families to discuss the trade-offs that result from approval of medications with substantial ongoing uncertainty about benefits to better represent the full range of views on this important question.

The committee recognizes the robust work of the public–private partnerships launched under Section 3 of the ACT for ALS: (1) CP-RND, (2) AMP ALS, and (3) ALL ALS. While these initiatives were being designed and priorities being set at the time of this report's writing, the committee offers the following recommendation for opportunities to be included in the developing priorities for ALS translational research:

Recommendation 5-2: Expand ALS translational research.

The ALS-focused public–private partnerships created under the Accelerating Access for Critical Therapies for ALS Act should consider additional translational research priorities that would accelerate therapeutic developments in ALS. The National Institutes of Health and the National Institute of Neurological Disorders and Stroke should prioritize ALS research including the following:

   a. **Understand the staging of disease, for both familial and sporadic ALS, in particular the preclinical disease or prodromal state, to inform when to intervene with therapeutics.**
   b. **Create and sustain a comprehensive, robust, and indefinitely ongoing natural history study across diverse patient populations and different stages of disease that could serve as external and concurrent controls for some clinical trials. This could help reduce the number of placebo-controlled designs for early phase trials and longer treatment duration clinical trials.**

   c. Develop additional validated biomarkers that would enable identifying and monitoring disease progression, including the early molecular and cellular changes hypothesized to occur before the appearance of clinical symptoms, and to monitor effects of therapeutic interventions (e.g., TDP-43 pathology).

   d. Advance the identification of new therapeutic targets derived from a better understanding of the pathophysiology of sporadic ALS, including an understanding of plateaus when ALS disease progression stops or slows significantly for a period of time.

   e. Advance novel drug delivery methods and ALS patient-friendly formulations that are safe, effective, and allow greater inter-dose intervals and flexibility for ALS individuals with dysphagia, intravenous access, or lumbar puncture difficulties.

   f. Engage diverse stakeholders and experts with a variety of viewpoints and support research regarding the trade-offs between having new products to try, even absent compelling evidence of meaningful benefit, and developing safe and effective drugs for treating and preventing ALS and to improve the use of the expanded access pathway to ease the tension in demanding earlier drug approvals.

ESTABLISHING A COMPREHENSIVE ALS REGISTRY

In the committee's view, a robust registry of people with ALS is a necessary tool to measure progress toward making ALS a more livable disease. It would collect data on care, outcomes, and risk factors, providing a valuable population-level perspective on living with ALS. This data would be collected as a routine part of care. The committee considered how best to expand the Centers for Disease Control and Prevention's (CDC's) already-existing National ALS Registry to meet that goal.

ALS data collection today is fragmented and uncoordinated. Different types of data in various formats exist in registries, individual academic centers, researchers' labs, and at the more than 50 ALS nonprofit organizations operating across the United States. These dispersed and fragmented efforts raise the costs for individual projects, limit their ability to test multiple hypotheses, and restrict their capability to track the size and health of the overall ALS population. Establishing a comprehensive ALS registry is a key opportunity to address this problem.

Patient registries can be a powerful source of real-world disease data. When properly designed and implemented, registries can provide an accurate picture of clinical practice, patient outcomes, safety, and disease epidemiology. Depending on their design, rare disease patient registries can help researchers follow the disease's natural history, track progress at the population level, recruit people into clinical trials, and accomplish other key goals such as determining whether earlier diagnosis, new therapeutics, or improvements in the care process are improving outcomes for people with the disease as a whole (Mayberry and McCleary, 2016; McGettigan et al., 2019) (see Box 5-2 for the difference between a registry and natural history study). For example, a recent analysis of the Irish population-based ALS registry revealed that despite changes in ALS care over the past 25 years, widespread use of noninvasive ventilation, and aggressive secretion management, as well as the overall increased incidence and prevalence of ALS in Ireland, the survivability of ALS has not improved (McFarlane et al., 2023).

A critical role of registries is to provide a population-level view of a disease. By doing so, registries can offer insights into the accessibility or quality of care, the distribution of known and potential risk factors,

---

BOX 5-2
Registries and Natural History Studies

A registry is a system for collecting, storing, analyzing, and disseminating information in a standardized format on individuals with a disease, who are predisposed to its occurrence, or who have been exposed to known or suspected causative environmental factors. A registry may be used to collect disease information, recruit patients for clinical trials, monitor patient care and outcomes, advance research hypotheses, observe patient behavior patterns, establish disease-specific standards of care, and support reimbursement discussions. Registries can be used as a source of data or enrollment for natural history studies.

Natural history studies are designed with a specific intent, such as tracking the course of a disease over time; identifying variables that correlate with the disease and outcomes in the absence of treatment, including demographics, environmental conditions, and genetic variables; and informing clinical trial design. Natural history studies document the disease's course from the time immediately prior to inception, progressing from the presymptomatic phase through various clinical stages to the time when the patient is cured, becomes chronically disabled, or dies in the absence of clinical intervention. Natural history studies can also generate information about how a disease develops and provide clues on possible therapeutic approaches.

SOURCE: O'Brien, 2022.

and overall progress in survivability These questions can be further disaggregated by race, ethnicity, income level, insurance status, and other demographic data to assess the resources and difficulties of different populations.

Registries also offer a potential avenue for recruiting people with a disease into clinical trials. Registry enrollment can help researchers identify large numbers of potential subjects to participate in clinical trials (Tan et al., 2015). The NIH-funded Rare Disease Clinical Research Network, for example, launched a contact registry specifically to connect patients and researchers to advance rare disease research. In addition, registries can show the community what research is ongoing. Many registries maintain a public list of research using their data (Mayberry and McCleary, 2016). Not only does this encourage people with the disease to participate in the registry, but it also serves as another method to connect interested members of the community with researchers. Demonstrating the effects of research can also encourage philanthropic funders to invest more in relevant grants or organizations. When possible, epidemiological data from a registry should be linked to other data sources, such as biorepositories.

A Comparable Registry

Patient registries have been used to great effect in other disease spaces, such as cystic fibrosis. Cystic fibrosis affects close to 40,000 children and adults of every racial and ethnic population in the United States. The Cystic Fibrosis Foundation (CFF) established the CFF Patient Registry (CFFPR) in the 1960s to collect information on patient demographics and survival. Today, the registry serves as an important source of information for research, clinical care, and tracking incidence, survival, and population trends regarding cystic fibrosis and related disorders (Knapp et al., 2016).[6]

CFFPR enrolls all individuals diagnosed with cystic fibrosis and associated disorders seen at one of the 121 CFF-accredited care centers and 51 affiliate programs across the United States and who provide informed consent. Data is collected primarily from clinical reports and assessments generated as a standard part of care, though other sources such as electronic medical records and U.S. Census data are linked as well. During the course of care, CFF staff input the data via an online registry portal. Every CFF-accredited clinic must participate in the registry, and a portion of each center's CFF funding is based on the number of patients enrolled in the registry and the completeness of these records.

---

[6]Cystic fibrosis transmembrane conductance regulator (CFTR) related metabolic syndrome and other CFTR-related disorders.

Every CFF clinic's institutional review board (IRB) must approve the CFFPR's data collection and use protocols annually, with CFF's privacy counsel providing additional oversight. A CFF committee and external experts must approve individual requests to access CFFPR data, and CFF has strict publication and data destruction policies for any researcher who is using identifiable data. Data are further protected by institutional information technology policies; CFF maintains the registry's data on a secure platform that meets FDA standards for data integrity and the standards of the Health Information Technology for Economic Clinical Health Act.

Today, clinical care teams use the CFF registry for pre-visit planning and patient care management. Health care systems use the registry to examine center-level variation in treatment and care practices and evaluate quality improvement initiatives, and researchers use the registry to obtain annual estimates of incidence, prevalence, mortality, and secondary complications; conduct natural history studies; and to gain insights on the etiology of disease (CFF, 2023; Comeau et al., 2004).

The Existing National ALS Registry

The CDC National ALS Registry, launched in October 2010, is the primary nationwide effort to count ALS cases in the United States. (Box 5-3 describes the data the National ALS Registry collects, as well as important information that it does not collect.) Using the most recently available data, CDC estimated there were 29,824 people living with ALS in the United States in 2018 (Mehta et al., 2023). This estimate is based off a count of 21,665 definite cases identified via Medicare, Veterans Health Administration, and Veterans Benefits Administration databases, as well as an online portal for self-identification and statistical modeling (Mehta et al., 2023). Based on an estimate of new cases identified in 2018 in administrative databases and CDC's patient portal, it is estimated that these methods missed approximately 27 percent of cases (Mehta et al., 2023).

CDC records demographic information for all registrants via self-enrollment or administrative data. Individuals with ALS provide other information, such as clinical characteristics and risk factor exposure, via optional National ALS Registry risk factor surveys. After initial enrollment, people with ALS in the registry are given the option via email to complete or update these surveys via the registry's online portal. Enrollees are also asked to complete the disease progression survey, which asks enrollees to report their ALSFRS-R score every 3 months after enrollment, and again, completing this survey is optional. After 1 year of enrollment, enrollees are asked to update their functional rating every 6 months. Notification for other surveys is sent every 6 months.

BOX 5-3
National ALS Registry Data Needs

Variables available for all registry participants include:

- Age range at diagnosis
- Year of diagnosis
- Sex
- City and state of residence at diagnosis
- Race

Data currently collected by the National ALS Registry that should be more routinely collected:

- Presence or absence of various environmental factors
- Use of pharmacological and nonpharmacological interventions
- Participation in biorepositories or other registries, with data linkages as appropriate

Data not currently collected by the National ALS Registry:

- Time to diagnosis
- Time from symptom onset to diagnosis and/or death
- Patient-centered clinical outcomes beyond ALSFRS-R score
- Equity and quality-of-life measures
- Care factors, such as where the person with ALS receives care

---

Gaps in the National ALS Registry

As it currently exists, the National ALS Registry is inadequate regarding several key pieces of information, including:

- Completeness: Several evaluations suggest that counts based on administrative databases and self-identification alone miss a significant portion of people living with ALS in the United States (Kaye et al., 2018; Nelson et al., 2021; Raymond et al., 2023). Risk factor surveys have also had low response rates (Bryan et al., 2016; Raymond et al., 2021).
- Representativeness: National ALS Registry data are not representative of the United States population as a whole, particularly in terms of people of color with ALS, younger people with ALS, and

- Identity and relationship of primary caregiver
- Development of comorbid conditions, such as frontotemporal dementia
- Genetic status

Variables only available for some registry participants include:

- History of military service
- Smoking and alcohol consumption
- ALSFRS-R score
- Physical activity
- Family history of ALS and other neurological diseases
- Clinical data (e.g., devices used, body onset, clinical symptoms)
- Year of symptom onset
- Site of symptom onset
- Lifetime residential history
- Lifetime occupational history
- Residential pesticide use
- Head and neck injuries
- Caffeine consumption
- Hobbies with toxicants
- Hormonal and reproductive history
- Pharmacological and nonpharmacological interventions

SOURCE: National ALS Registry, 2024.

people with ALS with private health insurance (Kaye et al., 2018; Nelson et al., 2021; Raymond et al., 2023).

- Date of diagnosis: This is only captured based on patient recall; without knowing the true date of diagnosis, incidence data cannot be accurately calculated. Some researchers have opted against using date of diagnosis as an endpoint due to this recall bias (Bryan et al., 2016).
- Timeliness: Because it takes a long time to procure and process administrative claims data, the data in the National ALS Registry are not current enough to maximize their effect; recent CDC prevalence studies have been based on 5-year-old data (Mehta, 2023). Without more current data, it is impossible to track the population-level effects of advances in care, therapeutics, and access.

Other patient registries—CFFPR, the Swedish Motor Neuron Disease Quality Registry,[7] and other national and regional European ALS registries, for example—have achieved high rates of completeness when compared to the nationwide prevalence of their respective diseases. Though these registries are constructed under different circumstances than CDC's National ALS Registry, they still offer useful insights. For example, CFF bases a portion of a care center's funding on the number of patients it enrolls in the registry and the completeness of the data for those patients (Faro, 2024). This suggests that robust linkages between individual ALS clinics and the National ALS Registry may incentivize improved data collection. Similarly, differences between national health care systems may make it more likely people living with ALS in other countries receive care at a specialty clinic, or those nations' health data may be centralized in a national resource suggesting that improved access to registration (and, more broadly, quick diagnosis and specialty ALS care) is important for producing a more complete registry (Abhinav et al., 2007). Finally, some international ALS registries do rely on voluntary enrollment, suggesting that high ascertainment rates can be achieved with that method (Walker et al., 2019; Wolfson et al., 2023).

The National ALS Registry's Role in the ALS Data Landscape

As noted in Chapter 1, many efforts across the ALS landscape developed concurrently with this study. Several of these are working to collect data regarding people with ALS. The National ALS Registry remains the primary effort to collect risk factor data and population statistics for ALS, and this report's recommendations seek to expand that role. However, there are other useful types of data being collected by laboratories, nonprofits, and research consortia; it is important that these data not remain siloed. To best serve the research needs related to ALS, the National ALS Registry should achieve interoperability with these other data sources. Data elements and definitions should be aligned as much as possible, and opportunities to link data in the National ALS Registry to that of other sources should be realized.

Biorepositories

Biorepositories collect fluids and tissue from people with a disease pre- or post-mortem; these can help researchers answer questions about the biology of a disease. Several groups already maintain biorepositories

---

[7]Motor neuron disease (MND) is a category of disease of which ALS is the most common. Many European research, registry, and advocacy efforts for MND focus largely on ALS, and the term is used somewhat interchangeably.

for ALS, including CDC, whose National ALS Biorepository is connected to its registry. This suggests existing potential for further connections between the National ALS Registry and other biorepositories. Other biorepositories include those maintained by Target ALS, the VA, and NEALS. Under the ACT for ALS, NINDS is also standing up a nationwide ALS clinical research consortium called ALL ALS. While ALL ALS is still in its design phase, its biorepository and research portfolio will be focused on identifying biomarkers for ALS.

When researchers know more about the people from whom these samples came, they are better able to design studies and make conclusions to answer questions of scientific interest; linking to a registry would provide this information. The National ALS Registry should allow for centrally linking sample information to individual cases of ALS.

State ALS Registries

A few states have or are in the process of establishing their own state-level registries with mandatory reporting requirements. Massachusetts was the first state to establish its own ALS registry and required health care providers to report ALS patient data annually to the registry (Raymond et al., 2023). In May 2022, both Vermont and Maine passed legislation creating a state registry and mandated reporting, and California followed suit in October 2023. California's registry will also include entries for other neurodegenerative diseases.

Ideally, the National ALS Registry would be a single, comprehensive registry containing data on all people living with ALS in the United States, as well as genetic carriers. Its data would go beyond epidemiological measures; an ideal ALS registry would include population-level data necessary to track and improve care for people living with ALS. However, the committee recognizes the current resource challenges faced by the National ALS Registry as is, as well as the time and investment necessary to increase the scope of the registry.

Until a single, more complete and comprehensive ALS registry is more feasible, the National ALS Registry should be built to be interoperable with state ALS registries. Data from state registries should be regularly reported to CDC, and these registries should use similar infrastructures and definitions.

At-Risk Genetic Carriers and the National ALS Registry

A more complete discussion of at-risk genetic carriers for ALS, as well as how to further prevent ALS in this population, can be found in Chapter 6. However, a comprehensive National ALS Registry should allow at-risk genetic carriers to enroll. This would allow for a more comprehensive count of the prevalence of genes related to familial ALS and of the incidence of ALS in at-risk carriers.

Including at-risk genetic carriers in the registry would also help researchers understand the development of familial ALS. For example, a comprehensive registry could capture data on risk and protective factors for people with various ALS-associated genes. It could also capture more robust population health data over time, such as on when and how often people with certain genes develop ALS (i.e., its penetrance). When at-risk genetic carriers do develop ALS, the registry would then continue to track them through their care journey. This would generate real-world data on how people with familial ALS progress through the disease and respond to care, given their genetic profile. Registry data could also inform future research into at-risk genetic carriers, such as natural history studies and prevention studies.

Reportability of ALS

ALS is not currently included in CDC's National Notifiable Conditions List. National Notifiable Conditions, also known as reportable diseases, are those for which cases are reported to CDC. CDC and the Council of State and Territorial Epidemiologists create the list of National Notifiable Conditions. While there is no legal mandate behind the list, state and local laws specify which conditions must be reported to their health departments, and most of the National Notifiable Conditions are universally reportable at the state and local level. These conditions are typically communicable diseases, such as botulism, cholera, COVID-19, and hepatitis. However, certain non-infectious conditions are also notifiable, such as cancer, elevated blood lead levels, and pesticide-related illness and injury (Thomas et al., 2017).

There is enough evidence to support the idea that environmental factors play a crucial role in the development of ALS, and the only way to reliably identify and mitigate these risks is through a comprehensive registry that includes every individual in the nation who is diagnosed with ALS. Until ALS is a mandated notifiable disease nationwide, it will be impossible to know the true prevalence or incidence of ALS and when the disease becomes livable or survivable at the population level.

Privacy Concerns

Storing the personal information of people with ALS, as would be necessary for a registry, naturally raises privacy concerns, especially if ALS becomes a reportable disease at the state and territorial levels. People with ALS and their families may be concerned that enrollment in a registry may open the door to discrimination. Information about genetic discrimination related to ALS can be found in Chapter 6. However, this concern may be broader. While laws exist to protect against discrimination based on health status, the best way to alleviate this concern is for the National ALS Registry to include a robust set of privacy and confidentiality protections.

The National ALS Registry already has several such protections in place. Sensitive data fields are hidden during enrollment on CDC's web portal, data are encrypted, and personally identifiable information is moved daily to a secure database with no internet access. Moreover, CDC requires IRB approval from the institution of any researcher seeking to access National ALS Registry data. These policies should be expanded as the use of registry data for research also grows. Peer registries such as the CFFPR may be a useful model. Committees of both CFF and academic experts review all external requests for data, and data-sharing agreements typically include publication and data destruction policies.

Further exploration of information technology policies may also help ensure the security of registry data, especially as registry data is made more available to clinicians. Examples include regular third-party risk evaluations; a least-privileges access framework, which limits the amount of information available to end users to what is strictly necessary; verifying the security of its web portals, pursuant to NIH data protection rules; and pursuing an NIH Certificate of Confidentiality, which certifies the privacy of research participants and limits disclosure of identifiable information.

In the absence of a comprehensive national registry of ALS, meaningful assessments of overall trends in the health of people with ALS are impossible. A comprehensive registry of people with ALS is a necessary tool to measure progress toward making ALS a more livable disease. The committee offers the following recommendation to ensure that a comprehensive registry is created as part of a larger ALS data platform, which should be strengthened by requiring clinicians to report all cases of ALS nationally.

Recommendation 5-3: Build a comprehensive ALS registry as part of a larger ALS data platform.

The Centers for Disease Control and Prevention (CDC) and the National Institute of Neurological Disorders and Stroke (e.g., ALL ALS consortium) should integrate new and current data sources with CDC's National ALS Registry to create a comprehensive, interoperable data platform capable of collecting detailed, geocoded, longitudinal data on all individuals living with ALS, as well as people at increased genetic risk of developing ALS. To make this registry most useful, CDC and the Council of State and Territorial Epidemiologists should add ALS to the National Notifiable Diseases Surveillance System, and states should require clinicians report all cases of ALS.

All accredited ALS care centers should also be required to participate in the National ALS Registry, with a portion of supplemental funding for a center based on the number of patients enrolled in the registry and the completeness of these records, as is done for CFF's patient registry. A comprehensive National ALS Registry should be embedded in routine ALS care; every person with ALS receiving care at a multidisciplinary clinic should be automatically enrolled into the registry. This would allow the registry to collect necessary data for answering key population health questions. Box 6-3 describes types of data not currently collected by the National ALS Registry that would be useful to answer such questions. While people with ALS may individually choose not to disclose such information, they may not opt out of being counted. Even if a person with ALS does not have an individual entry in the registry, counting them is important to measure overall prevalence and incidence of the disease, as is done for other notifiable conditions.

The National ALS Registry should report this data back to clinics, as is done with peer registries such as the CFF Patient Registry. This would allow multidisciplinary clinics to assess the quality of the care they deliver. It may also inform research, such as into local environmental risk factors or access to care. Reporting should be based on as recent data as is feasible; the current 5-year delay seen in National ALS Registry publications reduces its usefulness for the ALS community. Finally, this registry should be linked to other key data sources, such as those maintained by nonprofits and research consortia, to create a comprehensive data platform tracking all facets of ALS at the population level.

NEW AND EMERGING
NONPHARMACOLOGICAL TECHNOLOGIES

Technological advances in robotics, sensing technologies, virtual reality, and artificial intelligence have introduced many opportunities for technology-mediated tools that may provide support for persons with ALS and their families and improve their quality of life at home. For example, advances in telehealth technology have accelerated home monitoring opportunities, such as video conferencing to support virtual visits with clinicians, capturing vital signs, remotely assessing gait and balance, and capture activities of daily living and sleep quality. Online communities and caregiver support apps are already available and provide access to information, connection among peers, and creating virtual networks.

The committee notes that emerging technologies should be developed with engagement from end users, consideration of data privacy and security, attention to inclusive technologies that reduce health disparities, and using technology to facilitate and increase access to clinical trials for individuals living with ALS. This section also discusses reimbursement considerations related to emerging technologies.

Communication

Eye-tracking communication devices enable people with advanced paralysis to communicate using eye movements, providing a lifeline for expression and interaction (Caligari et al., 2013). Brain–computer interfaces (BCIs) allow patients to communicate by translating brain signals into text or speech, offering an alternative communication method for those with severe motor impairments (Vlek et al., 2012). In early 2014, one group of investigators had demonstrated that most severely disabled people with ALS could use the Wadsworth BCI (P300-based) home system (McCane et al., 2014). More recently, researchers recruited people living with ALS who are unable to communicate verbally or through writing to assess the functional reliability and extent of use of the Wadsworth BCI home system for communication, using email and audio/video programs (Wolpaw et al., 2018). The system was reliable and useful, and according to most patients and caregivers, using BCI introduced benefits that outweighed any burdens or challenges associated with its use.

Mobility

Robotic exoskeletons aid in mobility and enhance independence by assisting with walking and performing daily activities (Tanabe et al., 2013). Exoskeletons offer a safe and convenient approach to neurorehabilitation that does not cause physical exhaustion and imposes minimal demands on cognitive resources. Learning to operate an exoskeleton is straightforward, and they enhance mobility, enhance overall function, and decrease the likelihood of secondary injuries by restoring a more natural walking pattern. However, a challenge in this field lies in the absence of established experimental methods for assessing the comparative effectiveness of exoskeletons compared to other rehabilitation methods and technologies.

Controlling the Environment

Individuals with ALS have successfully operated a robot using a joystick and buttons to navigate around obstacles, pick up objects with various configurations and across different types of flooring, and deliver them to the individual (King et al., 2012). Another system that allowed people with ALS to control a wheelchair using their eyes received high overall satisfaction scores from individuals with ALS (Elliott et al., 2019). This innovative technology does not rely on preserved motor function or speech but solely on oculomotor function. Versatile robotic systems have the potential not only to assist patients but also to play a role in their evaluation, training, and ongoing assessment, all within the same robotic framework.

Smart home technologies using passive sensing, such as with motion and light sensors, can provide information about residents' well-being, detect emergencies, and even allow remote control of lighting and temperature. In some instances, machine learning can enable these technologies to "learn" the habits and preferences of residents, families, and visitors and provide an adaptive environment as health care needs change. One group of investigators used BCI components linked to a smart home system that allowed users to control home devices such as lamps, blinds, webcams, and telephones (Gao et al., 2018).

Reimbursement for Emerging Technologies

One of the things that I have experienced is most people that get ALS tend to be older, and so the doctors and companies I have worked with almost seem like, why do you need access for your wheelchair to be used with, for example, computer equipment and a mouse? I'm still pretty young and still pretty techy so I would like to be able to access those things, and I feel that it has been difficult to get support in that way.

—Julian Rodriguez, person living with ALS, presented during August 2023 public workshop

Health insurance reimbursement for medical devices supporting people with ALS is complex and variable. Depending on the carrier, insurance companies may cover respiratory support devices, assistive communication technology, and mobility equipment. Reimbursement eligibility is determined by varying insurance plan policies and provider documentation of medical necessity. In general Medicare will cover 80 percent of the cost to purchase or rent covered durable medical equipment, including walkers, wheelchairs, patient lifts, bilevel positive airway pressure (BiPAP) machines, speech-generating devices, and hospital beds. In the case of most evolving technologies, even when covered, people living with ALS face the same reimbursement challenges as with more traditional medical devices.

There is progress, however. In 2024, the Centers for Medicare & Medicaid Services (CMS) provided coverage under the Medicare brace benefit category for a robotic exoskeleton for neurologic injuries. Previously, gait-assist exoskeletons were covered by some commercial payers on a case-by-case basis. Recently, CMS added RelieVRx, a virtual reality device for treating chronic lower back pain, to its durable medical equipment category. More broadly, in 2023, CMS announced a proposed Transitional Coverage for Emerging Technologies pathway to provide an efficient review process for FDA-designated Breakthrough Devices.

Coverage policies for emerging technologies are largely determined by validation of clinical efficacy derived from clinical research studies.

Because findings may also apply to patients with strokes, traumatic brain injury, spinal cord disorders, and Parkinson's disease, it may be possible to conduct larger studies with a wider range of patients. Ultimately, funding of these studies is critical to receive not only FDA approval but also third-party reimbursement.

> **Recommendation 5-4: Fund neglected areas of research that would yield near-term gains in quality of life for people with ALS.**

The National Institutes of Health (NIH), the National Institute of Neurological Disorders and Stroke (NINDS), the Agency for Healthcare Research and Quality (AHRQ), and other ALS research funders should prioritize research to learn what works best in ALS care and increase support for other critical areas of ALS research that are currently neglected but would yield near-term gains in quality of life for persons with ALS. NIH, NINDS, AHRQ, and other ALS research funders should prioritize ALS research to include the following:

a. Research health services and evaluate nonpharmacologic interventions, services, and models that can provide a high quality of life for individuals living with ALS, such as large, prospective studies of rehabilitative therapy interventions including physical therapy, speech and language supports, and respiratory therapy.

b. Support social and behavioral research to determine the areas of intervention at the intersection of clinical care and social connections.

c. Promote research of ALS biology and protective factors, including how ALS spreads in the body, why there are slow and fast progressors, why some people with ALS experience a plateau where symptoms remain stable, and why some individuals develop ALS only in one limb.

d. Determine how ALS develops following trauma.

e. Develop better clinical outcomes of function, survival prediction, and quality of life.

f. Develop emerging technologies focused on end user needs to better assist individuals living with ALS with functionality in their homes and improve overall quality of life.

g. Apply artificial intelligence (AI) in electronic medical records to help clinicians recognize the symptoms of ALS early on and refer individuals to an ALS specialist for diagnosis. In addition, use AI in search engines to help individuals explore symptoms they experience that might indicate they have ALS and prompt them to seek medical advice.

REFERENCES

Abhinav, K., B. Stanton, C. Johnston, J. Hardstaff, R. W. Orrell, R. Howard, J. Clarke, M. Sakel, M. A. Ampong, C. E. Shaw, P. N. Leigh, and A. Al-Chalabi. 2007. Amyotrophic lateral sclerosis in south-east England: A population-based study. The South-East England Register for Amyotrophic Lateral Sclerosis (SEALS Registry). *Neuroepidemiol* 29(1–2):44–48.

Adaptive Clinical Trials Coalition. 2019. Adaptive platform trials: Definition, design, conduct and reporting considerations. *Nature Reviews. Drug Discovery* 18(10):797–807.

ALS TDI (ALS Therapeutic Development Institute). 2022. Eledon announces phase 2a trial results for tegoprubart—A drug invented at ALS TDI. In *ALS TDI blog*. Watertown, MA: ALS Therapeutic Development Institute.

ALS TDI. 2024. *ALS Research Collaborative: Unlocking the power of data and collaboration to end ALS*. https://www.als.net/arc (accessed May 24, 2024).

Answer ALS. 2024. *IPS cells & motor neurons*. https://www.answerals.org/ips-cells-motor-neurons (accessed May 24, 2024).

Berger, A., M. Locatelli, X. Arcila-londono, G. Hayat, N. Olney, J. Wymer, K. Gwathmey, C. Lunetta, T. Heiman-Patterson, S. Ajroud-Driss, E. A. Macklin, M. A. Bind, K. Goslin, T. Stuchiner, L. Brown, T. Bazan, T. Regan, A. Adamo, V. Ferment, C. Schroeder, M. Somers, G. Manousakis, K. Faulconer, E. Sinani, J. Mirochnick, H. Yu, A. V. Sherman, and D. Walk. 2023. The natural history of ALS: Baseline characteristics from a multi-center clinical cohort. *Amyotroph Lateral Scler Frontotemporal Degener* 1–9.

Berry, J. D., R. Miller, D. H. Moore, M. E. Cudkowicz, L. H. Van den Berg, D. A. Kerr, Y. Dong, E. W. Ingersoll, and D. Archibald. 2013. The Combined Assessment of Function and Survival (CAFS): A new endpoint for ALS clinical trials. *Amyotroph Lateral Scler Frontotempor Degener* 14(3):162–168.

Bryan, L., W. Kaye, V. Antao, P. Mehta, O. Muravov, and D. K. Horton. 2016. Preliminary results of national amyotrophic lateral sclerosis (ALS) registry risk factor survey data. *PLoS One* 11(4):e0153683.

Caligari, M., M. Godi, S. Guglielmetti, F. Franchignoni, and A. Nardone. 2013. Eye tracking communication devices in amyotrophic lateral sclerosis: Impact on disability and quality of life. *Amyotroph Lateral Scler Frontotemporal Degener* 14(7–8):546–552.

Cedarbaum, J. M., N. Stambler, E. Malta, C. Fuller, D. Hilt, B. Thurmond, and A. Nakanishi. 1999. The ALSFRS-R: A revised ALS functional rating scale that incorporates assessments of respiratory function. BDNF ALS study group (Phase III). *J Neurol Sci* 169(1–2):13–21.

CIB (Center for Innovation & Bioinformatics). *ALS/Motor Neuron Disease (MND) Natural History Consortium*. https://www.data4cures.org/natural-history-consortium (accessed May 24, 2024).

CFF (Cystic Fibrosis Foundation). 2023. *Cystic fibrosis foundation patient registry 2022 annual data report*. Bethesda, MD.

Collignon, O., A. Schritz, R. Spezia, and S. J. Senn. 2021. Implementing historical controls in oncology trials. *Oncologist* 26(5):e859–e862.

Comeau, A. M., R. B. Parad, H. L. Dorkin, M. Dovey, R. Gerstle, K. Haver, A. Lapey, B. P. O'Sullivan, D. A. Waltz, R. G. Zwerdling, and R. B. Eaton. 2004. Population-based newborn screening for genetic disorders when multiple mutation DNA testing is incorporated: A cystic fibrosis newborn screening model demonstrating increased sensitivity but more carrier detections. *Pediatrics* 113(6):1573–1581.

C-Path (Critical Path Institute). 2024. *Critical path for rare neurodegenerative diseases*. https://c-path.org/program/critical-path-for-rare-neurodegenerative-diseases (accessed May 24, 2024).

Elliott, M. A., H. Malvar, L. L. Maassel, J. Campbell, H. Kulkarni, I. Spiridonova, N. Sophy, J. Beavers, A. Paradiso, C. Needham, J. Rifley, M. Duffield, J. Crawford, B. Wood, E. J. Cox, and J. M. Scanlan. 2019. Eye-controlled, power wheelchair performs well for ALS patients. *Muscle Nerve* 60(5):513–519.

ENCALS (European Network to Cure ALS). 2024. *About ENCALS.* https://www.encals.eu/about-encals (accessed May 24, 2024).

Fang, T., G. Je, P. Pacut, K. Keyhanian, J. Gao, and M. Ghasemi. 2022. Gene therapy in amyotrophic lateral sclerosis. *Cells* 11(13).

Faro, A. 2023. *Lessons learned: The evolution of CF care.* Presentation to the committee.

FDA (U.S. Food and Drug Administration). 2019. *Amyotrophic lateral sclerosis: Developing drugs for treatment guidance for industry.* U.S. Department of Health and Human Services. https://www.fda.gov/media/130964/download (accessed April 11, 2024).

FDA-NIH (National Institutes of Health) Biomarker Working Group. 2016. *BEST (biomarkers, endpoints, and other tools) resource.* Silver Spring, MD, and Bethesda, MD: U.S. Food and Drug Administration and National Institutes of Health.

Gao, Q., X. Zhao, X. Yu, Y. Song, and Z. Wang. 2018. Controlling of smart home system based on brain-computer interface. *Technol Health Care* 26(5):769–783.

Ghadessi, M., R. Tang, J. Zhou, R. Liu, C. Wang, K. Toyoizumi, C. Mei, L. Zhang, C. Q. Deng, and R. A. Beckman. 2020. A roadmap to using historical controls in clinical trials—by Drug Information Association Adaptive Design Scientific Working Group (DIA-ADSWG). *Orphanet J Rare Dis* 15(1):69.

Jahanshahi, M., K. Gregg, G. Davis, A. Ndu, V. Miller, J. Vockley, C. Ollivier, T. Franolic, and S. Sakai. 2021. The use of external controls in FDA regulatory decision making. *Ther Innov Regul Sci* 55(5):1019–1035.

Katyal, N., and R. Govindarajan. 2017. Shortcomings in the current amyotrophic lateral sclerosis trials and potential solutions for improvement. *Front Neurol* 8:521.

Kaye, W. E., L. Wagner, R. Wu, and P. Mehta. 2018. Evaluating the completeness of the National ALS Registry, United States. *Amyotroph Lateral Scler Frontotemp Degener* 19(1–2):112–117.

King, C. H., T. L. Chen, Z. Fan, J. D. Glass, and C. C. Kemp. 2012. Dusty: An assistive mobile manipulator that retrieves dropped objects for people with motor impairments. *Disabil Rehabil Assist Technol* 7(2):168–179.

Knapp, E. A., A. K. H. Goss, A. Sewall, J. Ostrenga, C. Dowd, A. Elbert, K. M. Petren, and B. C. Marshall. 2016. The Cystic Fibrosis Foundation Patient Registry. Design and methods of a national observational disease registry. *Ann Am Thorac Soc* 13(7):1173–1179.

Mayberry, S. M., and K. McCleary. 2016. *Expanding the science of patient input: Building smarter patient registries.* Washington, DC: Milken Institute.

McCane, L. M., E. W. Sellers, D. J. McFarland, J. N. Mak, C. S. Carmack, D. Zeitlin, J. R. Wolpaw, and T. M. Vaughan. 2014. Brain-computer interface (BCI) evaluation in people with amyotrophic lateral sclerosis. *Amyotroph Lateral Scler Frontotempor Degener* 15(3–4):207–215.

McFarlane, R., C. Peelo, M. Galvin, M. Heverin, and O. Hardiman. 2023. Epidemiologic trends of amyotrophic lateral sclerosis in Ireland, 1996–2021. *Neurol* 101(19):e1905–e1912.

McGettigan, P., C. Alonso Olmo, K. Plueschke, M. Castillon, D. Nogueras Zondag, P. Bahri, X. Kurz, and P. G. M. Mol. 2019. Patient registries: An underused resource for medicines evaluation: Operational proposals for increasing the use of patient registries in regulatory assessments. *Drug Saf* 42(11):1343–1351.

Mead, R. J., N. Shan, H. J. Reiser, F. Marshall, and P. J. Shaw. 2023. Amyotrophic lateral sclerosis: A neurodegenerative disorder poised for successful therapeutic translation. *Nat Rev Drug Discov* 22(3):185–212.

Mehta, P., J. Raymond, Y. Zhang, R. Punjani, M. Han, T. Larson, O. Muravov, R. H. Lyles, and D. K. Horton. 2023. Prevalence of amyotrophic lateral sclerosis in the United States, 2018. *Amyotroph Lateral Scler Frontotempor Degener* 24(7–8):702–708.

Mishra-Kalyani, P. S., L. Amiri Kordestani, D. R. Rivera, H. Singh, A. Ibrahim, R. A. Declaro, Y. Shen, S. Tang, R. Sridhara, P. G. Kluetz, J. Concato, R. Pazdur, and J. A. Beaver. 2022. External control arms in oncology: Current use and future directions. *Ann Oncol* 33(4):376–383.

National ALS Registry. 2024. *Epidemiological/survey data requests.* https://www.cdc.gov/alsresearch/episurveydatarequests.html (accessed March 19, 2024).

NCRI (Neurological Clinical Research Institute). 2024. *Pooled resource open-access ALS clinical trials database.* https://ncri1.partners.org/ProACT/Document/DisplayLatest/5 (accessed May 24, 2024).

NEALS (Northeast Amyotrophic Lateral Sclerosis Consortium). 2024. https://neals.org/about/our-mission (accessed May 21, 2024).

Nelson, L. M., B. Topol, W. Kaye, J. Raymond, D. K. Horton, P. Mehta, and T. Wagner. 2021. Evaluation of the completeness of ALS case ascertainment in the US National ALS Registry: Application of the capture-recapture method. *Neuroepidemiol* 56(2):104–114.

NeuroNEXT (Network for Excellence in Neuroscience Clinical Trials). 2024. https://neuronext.org (accessed May 21, 2024).

NIH (National Institutes of Health). 2023. *Access for All in ALS (ALL ALS) East Clinical Coordinating Center.* https://reporter.nih.gov/project-details/10878218 (accessed May 21, 2024).

NINDS (National Institute of Neurological Disorders and Stroke). 2024. *Abnormal proteins found in the spinal fluid of people with ALS and frontotemporal dementia.* https://www.ninds.nih.gov/news-events/news/press-releases/abnormal-proteins-found-spinal-fluid-people-als-and-frontotemporal-dementia (accessed May 22, 2024).

O'Brien, K. 2022. *Leveraging registries and natural history studies to drive rare disease drug development.* https://acrpnet.org/2022/08/leveraging-registries-and-natural-history-studies-to-drive-rare-disease-drug-development (accessed April 11, 2024).

Quintana, M., B. R. Saville, M. Vestrucci, M. A. Detry, L. Chibnik, J. Shefner, J. D. Berry, M. Chase, J. Andrews, A. V. Sherman, H. Yu, K. Drake, M. Cudkowicz, S. Paganoni, and E. A. Macklin. 2023. Design and statistical innovations in a platform trial for amyotrophic lateral sclerosis. *Ann Neurol* 94(3):547–560.

Raymond, J., P. Mehta, T. Larson, E. P. Pioro, and D. K. Horton. 2021. Reproductive history and age of onset for women diagnosed with amyotrophic lateral sclerosis: Data from the national ALS registry: 2010–2018. *Neuroepidemiology* 55(5):416–424.

Raymond, J., R. Punjani, T. Larson, J. D. Berry, D. K. Horton, and P. Mehta. 2023. Comparing amyotrophic lateral sclerosis (ALS) patient characteristics from the National ALS Registry and the Massachusetts ALS Registry, data through 2015. *Amyotroph Lateral Scler Frontotemporal Degener* 1–8.

Seddighi, S., Y. A. Qi, A-L. Brown, O. G. Wilkins, C. Bereda, C. Belair, Y-J. Zhang, M. Prudencio, et al. 2024. Mis-spliced transcripts generate de novo proteins in TDP-43–related ALS/FTD. *Science Translational Medicine* 16(734).

Tan, M. H., M. Thomas, and M. P. Maceachern. 2015. Using registries to recruit subjects for clinical trials. *Contemp Clin Trials* 41:31–38.

Tanabe, S., S. Hirano, and E. Saitoh. 2013. Wearable power-assist locomotor (WPAL) for supporting upright walking in persons with paraplegia. *Neurorehabilit* 33(1):99–106.

Thomas, K., R. Jajosky, R. J. Coates, G. M. Calvert, D. Dewey-Mattia, J. Raymond, and S. D. Singh. 2017. Summary of notifiable noninfectious conditions and disease outbreaks: Surveillance data published between April 1, 2016, and January 31, 2017—United States. *Morb Mortal Wkly Rep* 64(54):1–6.

TRICALS (Treatment Research Initiative to Cure ALS). 2024. *About TRICALS: The highway towards a cure.* https://www.tricals.org/en/about (accessed May 24, 2024).

Vlek, R. J., D. Steines, D. Szibbo, A. Kübler, M. J. Schneider, P. Haselager, and F. Nijboer. 2012. Ethical issues in brain-computer interface research, development, and dissemination. *J Neurol Phys Ther* 36(2):94–99.

Walker, K. L., M. J. Rodrigues, B. Watson, C. Reilly, E. L. Scotter, H. Brunton, J. Turnbull, and R. H. Roxburgh. 2019. Establishment and 12-month progress of the New Zealand Motor Neurone Disease Registry. *J Clin Neurosci* 60:7–11.

Wolfson, C., D. E. Gauvin, F. Ishola, M. Oskoui, and B. Atabe. 2023. Epidemiological surveillance of amyotrophic lateral sclerosis: A review. *medRxiv* 2023.2011.2010.23297968.

Wolpaw, J. R., R. S. Bedlack, D. J. Reda, R. J. Ringer, P. G. Banks, T. M. Vaughan, S. M. Heckman, L. M. Mccane, C. S. Carmack, S. Winden, D. J. McFarland, E. W. Sellers, H. Shi, T. Paine, D. S. Higgins, A. C. Lo, H. S. Patwa, K. J. Hill, G. D. Huang, and R. L. Ruff. 2018. Independent home use of a brain-computer interface by people with amyotrophic lateral sclerosis. *Neurol* 91(3):e258–e267.

6

Preventing ALS

ABSTRACT

This chapter describes the challenge of identifying individuals at risk of developing amyotrophic lateral sclerosis (ALS) given the many genetic and environmental factors suspected of causing it. It discusses approaches for identifying at-risk individuals who harbor genes associated with the development of ALS and the research opportunities that arise from having larger numbers of such individuals, including the important role those individuals will play in identifying potential avenues to prevent ALS from developing. This chapter also addresses ethical and health communication challenges to conducting expanded carrier screening to identify asymptomatic carriers of ALS-associated gene mutations. These factors help explain how difficult preventing ALS is now and will continue to be for the near future. However, specific research approaches can help to mitigate these problems.

The key to preventing, halting, or reversing the characteristic nerve cell damage of ALS is identifying individuals at risk of developing the disease and then characterizing the genetic, biochemical, and environmental factors that trigger familial ALS and sporadic ALS (Benatar et al., 2023a). To achieve such a goal, the committee believes that focusing research on individuals at risk of developing ALS could provide important insights to enable halting or significantly slowing the development of ALS.

IDENTIFYING AT-RISK GENETIC CARRIERS

There are several possible approaches for identifying at-risk, presymptomatic individuals. For individuals who have a family history of the disease, genetic testing can identify those with mutations known to increase the risk of developing ALS. The Pre-symptomatic Familial ALS study (Pre-fALS) and PREVENT ALS study are examples of studies that build on this concept.[1] Both studies follow presymptomatic individuals with a family history of ALS to learn more about genetic and environmental factors that increase the risk of developing ALS (Benatar and Wuu, 2012; Benatar et al., 2023a; MGH, 2023).

While studying at-risk genetic carriers offers a critical opportunity to gain new insights into how, when, and why ALS develops, the challenge is to identify individuals with disease-causing or disease-moderating genes without a family history of ALS or who show no signs of developing ALS. Perhaps the only way to accomplish that on a scale large enough to be informative would be to conduct population-wide genetic screening, an approach that researchers have taken to identify asymptomatic genetic carriers for other diseases, including cancer, Lynch syndrome, and familial hypercholesterolemia (Grzymski et al., 2020; Nazareth et al., 2015). However, while rapidly falling costs of whole genome sequencing are making population-based screening more feasible logistically, there are several ethical and health communication challenges to conducting expanded carrier screening to identify asymptomatic carriers of ALS-associated gene mutations (ACOG Committee on Genetics, 2017; Evans et al., 2001; Oliveri et al., 2018; Roberts et al., 2020). These challenges include:

- The high emotional cost of genetic testing. There is a significant emotional burden for individuals who discover they harbor a genetic variation that could cause ALS in themselves as well as their children and grandchildren. There is also limited access to genetic counselors or mental health supports to help an individual cope with a genetic test result and interpret whether the genetic information is actionable.
- Complex family relationships when individuals within families have different perspectives on genetic testing. Some individuals will prefer to not know if they have a genetic mutation even if they had a family member with ALS. Individuals identified as genetic carriers may not know how to convey that information to

---

[1] Additional information is available at https://neals.org/als-trials/NCT00317616 (accessed June 10, 2024).

family members or may choose to not disclose that information to family members.

- Navigating the medical system with a confirmed genetic carrier status can be challenging since many clinicians are unsure of how to deal with an individual with a confirmed genetic risk for ALS. In addition, there are few guidelines for what to do after an individual has been identified as a genetic carrier (ACOG Committee on Genetics, 2017; AMA, n.d.).
- There is legitimate fear that an individual's genetic status could be used to deny insurance, services, or employment. While the Genetic Information Nondiscrimination Act (GINA) prohibits health insurers from discrimination based on genetic information, GINA's protections do not apply to life, disability, or long-term care insurance or to businesses with fewer than 15 employees (ASHG, 2008).

For the Pre-fALS study, the research team developed a set of principles and practices for ALS presymptomatic genetic testing. These include offering voluntary and informed consent, evaluating participants for psychosocial readiness, providing genetic counseling and information on testing logistics, providing predecision counseling to explore motivations for testing, and providing pretest and posttest counseling (Benatar et al., 2016).

One recent study using functional genomics combined with machine learning claims to have discovered 690 genes potentially associated with ALS (Zhang et al., 2022). Given these numbers, it is likely there are more individuals at risk of developing ALS who never develop the disease than there are people diagnosed with ALS. Several population-based modeling studies using methodology originally developed for cancer epidemiology suggest the development of ALS is a multistep process, which would mean that having an ALS-associated gene would not be sufficient by itself to cause ALS (Al-Chalabi et al., 2014; Chia et al., 2018; Vucic et al., 2019, 2020).

Identifying Factors Beyond Genetics

For the 90 percent of individuals who develop ALS without a family history of disease (Fang et al., 2022), and for individuals with genes known to be involved in familial ALS but do not develop the disease, research will need to identify other risk factors beyond inherited gene mutations, particularly environmental exposures, that elevate the risk of becoming symptomatic. For example, biological relatives of people with ALS without a known genetic basis have an eightfold increased risk of developing ALS (Hanby et al., 2011), and approximately 5 to 10 percent of individuals with frontotemporal dementia also develop ALS signs (Ferrari et al., 2011).

At the same time, about half of the first-degree relatives of individuals with ALS develop the disease, and studying those who do not develop ALS might provide insights into protective mechanisms (Ryan et al., 2019). Other populations with elevated risk of developing ALS include people with mild motor impairment (Benatar et al., 2022a); veterans, who have twice the risk of the general population of developing ALS (Beard et al., 2017); and those exposed to various yet-to-be-identified environmental risk factors, a presumed trigger implicated in most individuals with nongenetic ALS (Goutman and Feldman, 2020). Population-based studies have found that genetic factors account for only half of the variation in the risk of developing ALS (Ryan et al., 2019).

Another strategy for teasing out the mechanisms that cause ALS is to identify and study individuals at reduced risk for ALS. Research has shown, for example, that certain drugs used to treat hypertension, diabetes, and cardiovascular disease appear to reduce the risk of developing ALS by an unknown protective mechanism of action (Cui et al., 2022; Pfeiffer et al., 2020). Studies of individuals who experience a plateau in disease symptoms or whose symptoms improve or even resolve and those with mutations in genes associated with ALS who live to old age without developing ALS symptoms might also provide insights that could advance efforts to prevent the disease (Bedlack et al., 2016; Harrison et al., 2018).

Access to Genetic Testing and Counseling

It is important that people with ALS and at-risk genetic carriers for ALS be able to access genetic testing and counseling. For them, genetic testing could reveal useful information for navigating their ALS journey and for making important family and health care decisions. In addition, more people having access to their genetic information would provide more data for researchers seeking to answer the questions posed in earlier sections of this chapter.

Access to genetic testing and counseling for individuals living with ALS and their families varies widely. As discussed in Chapter 4, the level of services an ALS clinic can provide varies significantly across the country. Some clinics provide genetic testing and others do not. One study found that only 34.7 percent of people with ALS responding to an online survey were offered genetic testing during care (Wagner et al., 2017), while only 67.3 percent of those to whom genetic testing was offered undertook it. Almost 80 percent of respondents to the survey reported receiving care at a Muscular Dystrophy Association– and/or ALS Association (ALSA)-certified ALS clinic (Wagner et al., 2017). As a result, many individuals living with ALS have uncertain or limited access to genetic testing and counseling. Even when genetic testing is available, people with ALS may not be able to afford it given that the cost of such testing for all currently known genes associated with ALS is an estimated $6,000 (Vajda et al., 2017).

There are several methods by which people with ALS or at-risk genetic carriers might obtain genetic testing. Individuals living with ALS or at genetic risk of developing it who participate in clinical research will often receive free genetic testing as part of their participation in research. However, this only guarantees access to genetic testing for the approximately 10 percent of individuals living with ALS who participate in research and is not a sustainable solution (Mehta et al., 2021). ALSA has identified an opportunity for individuals living with ALS and their families to receive free genetic testing, sponsored by the biotechnology company, Biogen, and offered by Invitae, a genetic testing company.[2] The genetic testing panel looks for mutations in over 20 genes associated with ALS, including C9orf72. The duration of this program is unknown. The patient-led organization, Genetic ALS & FTD: End the Legacy, also includes information on genetic testing availability and guidance for accessing genetic counseling (End the Legacy, 2024).

Guidelines from professional associations and advisory boards has helped make genetic testing for other diseases more accessible. For example, the Affordable Care Act requires insurers to cover preventive services for which the U.S. Preventive Services Task Force (USPSTF) has issued an A or B rating, based on the evidence for its usefulness.[3] Both USPSTF and the National Cancer Center Network have recommended BRCA genetic testing for all women with certain family histories of cancer or BRCA inheritance.[4] In a 2018 survey, clinicians participating in the Northeast ALS Consortium reported they would offer genetic testing for individuals with ALS if guidelines for ALS existed (Klepek, 2018).

In September 2023, a group of ALS researchers and clinicians published a set of evidence-based consensus guidelines for the genetic testing and counseling of people with ALS (Roggenbuck et al., 2023). These guidelines call for testing every person with ALS for genes such as C9orf82, SOD1, FUS, and TARDBP; the publication also discussed genetic counseling guidelines. Groups such as ALSA have celebrated this development (ALSA, 2021). However, based on experiences in other disease spaces, such recommendations would be more powerful if they were included in ALS clinical practice guidelines, or if they were recommended by USPSTF.

---

[2]Additional information is available at https://ptcg.insideals.com/en-us/home/no-charge-genetic-testing.html (accessed June 10, 2024).

[3]See 29 CFR § 2590.715-2713 - Coverage of preventive health services.

[4]BReast CAncer gene.

Genetic Discrimination as a Barrier to Access

As noted above, at-risk genetic carriers for ALS may feel discouraged from pursuing genetic testing given the possibility of facing genetic discrimination when applying for insurance or a job. There are several protections in place for at-risk genetic carriers, but none are universal. For example, genetic information may be protected via standard research confidentiality processes. When an individual with a family history of ALS presents at an ALS clinic and requests genetic testing, it is not unusual for the clinic to refer the person to participate in a research study that includes provisions to safeguard the confidentiality of genetic test results, which includes keeping that information out of the individual's electronic health record.

There are also legal protections against genetic discrimination, the most notable of which is GINA.[5] GINA prohibits health insurers from asking about genetic information in many circumstances and from using genetic information to determine coverage eligibility or premiums. Employers with 15 or more employees have similar restrictions under GINA in that they may not use genetic information to make employment-related decisions. However, GINA does not prohibit genetic discrimination in life insurance, long-term care insurance, or disability insurance. These types of insurance are typically regulated by state legislatures, and there are a variety of factors to consider unique to each state's insurance market.

In light of the gaps and uncertainties around access to genetic testing and counseling, as well as the unresolved threat of genetic discrimination, the committee offers the following recommendation:

Recommendation 6-1: Increase access to genetic testing and counseling for people with ALS and their families.

Genetic testing and counseling should be made substantially more easily and consistently available for people with ALS and their families. The Centers for Medicare & Medicaid Services and private insurers should pay for genetic testing and counseling for all people living with ALS and their families. State legislatures should examine possible measures to prohibit genetic discrimination in life insurance, long-term care insurance, and disability insurance based on genetic risk for ALS.

Preventing ALS in At-Risk Genetic Carriers

There then is the case of individuals known to be at risk of developing ALS by virtue of their genetic makeup. Studying unaffected carriers of

---

[5]See Genetic Information Nondiscrimination Act of 2008, Public Law 110-233, 110th Congress (May 21, 2008).

pathogenic ALS variants has contributed to the development of a framework and initial lexicon for further study of the presymptomatic phase of ALS (Benatar et al., 2023b). The number of cohort studies comprising at-risk genetic carriers is growing, and the results may provide opportunities to investigate potential ALS prevention strategies and stimulate more natural history studies. This includes studies of biomarkers for developing ALS, such as neurofilament light chain protein (NfL). Some at-risk genetic carriers provide biological samples for ALS research multiple times, often gathered through invasive spinal fluid procedures, at different research sites across the country. The travel costs, lost wages, and emotional toll of this participation can be considerable. If an individual wishes to track their NfL levels as a potential marker of imminent phenoconversion, they must pay for it out of pocket.

There are also clinical trials evaluating the potential for preventing ALS. Tofersen, which the U.S. Food and Drug Administration (FDA) has approved as a treatment of ALS patients with SOD1 gene mutations, is the subject of the ATLAS trial, the first-ever ALS prevention trial.[6] The ATLAS study will monitor asymptomatic individuals with SOD1 mutations for increased blood levels of NfL. When levels of NfL rise above a predefined threshold, trial participants will be randomized to receive tofersen or placebo, to delay or even prevent the emergence of ALS symptoms (Benatar et al., 2022b). This type of clinical trial is complex and costly but will provide important data on the emergence of ALS.

Although involvement of the at-risk genetic carrier community in research is growing, many questions remain regarding how ALS develops in this population and whether it can be prevented with available or new drugs. It is unknown, for example, whether current FDA-approved therapeutics to treat ALS would be effective in delaying or preventing the onset of disease in at-risk genetic carriers. A September 2023 workshop involving clinicians, scientists, genetic counselors, and individuals with a genetic risk of developing ALS and frontotemporal dementia (FTD) explored the clinical science of treating and preventing ALS and FTD. Workshop participants are planning to draft recommendations and guidance for clinicians providing care for those at elevated risk of ALS and FTD (University of Miami, 2024).

Riluzole is currently being evaluated in at-risk genetic carriers who are willing to pay out of pocket both for clinic visits and for the drug (Abrevaya, 2023). The project seeks to determine if the onset of ALS symptoms can be delayed or prevented through early initiation of riluzole. The advocacy community points out the need for research on how ALS therapeutics work in genetic carriers before they develop ALS symptoms (End the

---

[6]Additional information is available at https://www.alsatlasstudy.com/en-us/home.html (accessed May 10, 2024).

Legacy, 2023). At-risk genetic carriers might be understandably interested in taking every possible step that might avoid the onset of ALS, including accessing ALS therapeutics before symptoms develop. The risk-benefit calculation is uncertain when considering dosing a healthy individual who may not develop ALS with therapeutics that include adverse side effects, such as elevated liver enzymes and interstitial pneumonia. In addition, a health insurer would likely object to paying for prescription ALS therapeutics in a healthy at-risk genetic carrier, leaving wealthier individuals with an advantage in trying these drugs if they can identify a clinician willing to prescribe.

Potential Preventive Therapies for Familial ALS

The most obvious kind of preventive intervention for familial ALS would be to delay or prevent disease gene expression, and some work has been done along these lines. Mutations in SOD1, C9orf72, TARDBP, and FUS genes are most associated with familial ALS. Mutations in the C9orf72 gene account for up to 40 percent of familial ALS in the United States and Europe (Nguyen et al., 2018). Worldwide, SOD1 gene mutations cause 12 to 20 percent of familial ALS and 1 to 2 percent of sporadic ALS (Amado and Davidson, 2021).

An antisense oligonucleotide targeting ATNX2 overproduction is in a Phase 1/2 trial, and jacifusen, an antisense oligonucleotide targeting the FUS mutation, has been investigated based on the drug's ability to virtually eliminate the toxic mutant FUS protein in the central nervous system (Korobeynikov et al., 2022). In 2021, the drug's developer started a Phase 3 trial that will enroll up to 64 people (Ray, 2021). Another antisense oligonucleotide, QRL-201, has begun Phase 1 trials; this agent restores function of stathmin-2, a protein required for nerve cell stability, the levels of which are affected by TDP-43 mutations. Two antisense oligonucleotides targeting C9orf72 overexpression completed Phase 1 clinical trials, but the trials' sponsors discontinued development of both of these agents when they demonstrated no clinical benefit despite reducing levels of toxic protein in cerebrospinal fluid (Biogen, 2022; Wave Life Sciences USA, 2023).

One approach that might delay or prevent the development of ALS would involve transplanting human neural progenitor cells into the spinal cord of people with or at risk of developing ALS. One Phase 1/2a study has shown that a single dose of human neural progenitor cells engineered to produce glial cell line-derived neurotrophic factor (GDNF) delivered into the lumbar spinal cord of 18 people with ALS had no negative effects at 1 year after injection (Baloh et al., 2022). Further study found that transplanted cells remained viable and continued to produce GDNF, which other research has shown can protect spinal motor neurons (Klein et al., 2005; Suzuki et al., 2007). Another Phase 1/2a proof-of-concept study is assessing the safety of injecting human neural progenitor cells engineered to produce GDNF into the motor cortex of people with ALS (Svendsen, 2023).

NONGENETIC FACTORS AND PREVENTION

Estimates of heritability, the extent of a disease attributable to genetics, in sporadic ALS vary from approximately 8.5 percent (van Rheenen et al., 2016) to approximately 61 percent (Al-Chalabi et al., 2010), suggesting contributions to ALS risk that go beyond genetics. Even for carriers of highly penetrant ALS mutations—those that result in ALS in most individuals with that mutation—onset occurs following a series of steps that may involve mutations in other genes or environmental exposures (Chiò et al., 2018). However, the emphasis of environmental studies in ALS have focused on the sporadic form, given the proportionately larger contribution of environmental exposures to disease risk in this category, and more prevention research focused on environmental exposures is needed in at-risk genetic carriers.

Investigation of environmental risk factors in ALS has given rise to the concept of the ALS exposome, the sum of environmental exposures over a lifetime that trigger disease onset (Goutman et al., 2023). Studies have aimed to characterize the ALS exposome and define the exposures that increase ALS risk. These efforts have identified a variety of potential exposures, including exposures to organic pollutants such as pesticides in the environment, metals, and air pollution; brain and spinal cord trauma; sports and intense physical activity; and possibly electromagnetic field exposure. The strength of the available evidence is well established for some of these exposures, such as certain pesticides (Goutman et al., 2023; Newell et al., 2022; Vasta et al., 2022).

Additional ALS risks may arise from occupational settings, such as manufacturing, construction, agriculture, and the military. For example, manufacturing and construction workers may be exposed to metal-containing welding fumes, volatile organic solvents, and particulate matter in exhaust fumes, whereas agricultural workers may be exposed to pesticides. Several recent studies demonstrate a connection between production occupations to ALS risk, as well as when and in what part of the body the disease first appears (Goutman et al., 2022a,b). Workers handling agriculture chemicals are also at elevated risk of developing ALS (Mitsumoto et al., 2022). In addition, exposure to toxins at home—if an individual's residence is next to agricultural fields or manufacturing plants that apply certain chemical pesticides with neurotoxic effects, for example—can also affect chances of developing the disease (Andrew et al., 2021).

Military personnel may be exposed to toxins while deployed in conflict zones or to trauma from mechanical injury to the brain or spinal cord that might lead to symptoms of ALS. In fact, strong evidence for a link between military service and ALS has existed for nearly 2 decades (IOM, 2006; McKay et al., 2021). However, basic research into the connection between military service and ALS has stalled in recent years. Improved researcher access to U.S. Department of Defense and U.S. Department of Veterans Affairs databases, along with longitudinal studies of these populations, would improve understanding of this connection.

Research on protective factors that could prevent the development of ALS has been limited. In the majority of instances, the mechanisms underlying ALS exposome-mediated neurodegeneration and triggering of ALS remain incompletely understood. A more comprehensive research program to fully delineate the ALS exposome and other risk factors could unlock the path to ALS prevention by removing or mitigating exposures.

The Need for Prospective ALS Studies

Many studies of the ALS exposome to date have been limited to retrospective studies using questionnaires to query past exposures. These research instruments are subject to recall bias, and, therefore, could limit study findings. Better characterization of the ALS exposome will require a prospective study design and querying exposures in real time, which is less subject to recall bias and generates more accurate information. Demographics, lifestyle, and clinical data can be collected in tandem, as can biospecimens for quantifying environmental exposures and biomarkers of neuronal damage. Populations at risk of ALS can be selected for these studies, because they are more likely to develop ALS, providing sufficient phenoconversion of individuals from health to disease to power prospective observations. Prospective, longitudinal studies of environmental risks should also include healthy individuals given that the causative factors for ALS are still unclear.

As the discussion in this chapter shows, involving at-risk genetic carriers in research would provide multiple avenues for investigating the causes of ALS and generating insights that could power the development of therapeutic or preventive agents. Other populations at risk of developing ALS also provide a valuable source of learning more about the environmental risks and deserve focused future study.

With the first prevention trial underway in an at-risk genetic carrier population (Biogen trial of tofersen) there is reason to believe additional research studies in genetic carriers will be possible in the future. To get to this point, the challenge is to develop evidence for clinical benefit and a biomarker signal in a symptomatic population before launching a study to evaluate disease progression or conversion to disease in an at-risk asymptomatic population. These studies can be long and challenging and will require increased collaboration and partnership among research funders, drug developers, and ALS nonprofit organizations and the affected communities to realize progress.

It is also the case that interventions are needed to prevent ALS not just for at-risk genetic carriers but also in sporadic ALS populations that may be at risk of developing ALS (e.g., veterans, football players). Risk identification is the first step, but risk mitigation approaches will need to be tested as interventions in clinical trials for at-risk individuals.

Therefore, the committee makes the following recommendation:

Recommendation 6-2: Advance research focused on populations at risk of developing ALS.

Research funders should partner with drug developers and the ALS community to advance research focused on populations at risk of developing ALS, including at-risk genetic carriers. Research funders should partner with drug developers and the ALS community to develop specific research programs focused on the unique unmet needs of at-risk genetic carriers. Research funders should support large-scale, prospective natural history studies of populations at risk of ALS.

REFERENCES

Abrevaya, S. 2023. *Synapticure launches an IRB-approved study for presymptomatic carriers of pathogenic, ALS-associated gene variants*. Chicago, IL: Synapticure.

ACOG (American College of Obstetricians and Gynecologists) Committee on Genetics. 2017. Committee opinion 690: Carrier screening in the age of genomic medicine. *Obstet Gynecol* 129(3):E35–E40.

Al-Chalabi, A., F. Fang, M. F. Hanby, P. N. Leigh, C. E. Shaw, W. Ye, and F. Rijsdijk. 2010. An estimate of amyotrophic lateral sclerosis heritability using twin data. *J Neurol Neurosurg Psychiatry* 81(12):1324–1326.

Al-Chalabi, A., A. Calvo, A. Chiò, S. Colville, C. M. Ellis, O. Hardiman, M. Heverin, R. S. Howard, M. H. B. Huisman, N. Keren, P. N. Leigh, L. Mazzini, G. Mora, R. W. Orrell, J. Rooney, K. M. Scott, W. J. Scotton, M. Seelen, C. E. Shaw, K. S. Sidle, R. Swingler, M. Tsuda, J. H. Veldink, A. E. Visser, L. H. Van Den Berg, and N. Pearce. 2014. Analysis of amyotrophic lateral sclerosis as a multistep process: A population-based modelling study. *Lancet Neurol* 13(11):1108–1113.

ALSA (ALS Assocation). 2021. *thinkALS™ for faster diagnosis*. https://www.als.org/thinkals (accessed April 5, 2024).

AMA (American Medical Association). n.d. *AMA Code of Medical Ethics: Genetic testing and counseling*. Chicago, IL: American Medical Association.

Amado, D. A., and B. L. Davidson. 2021. Gene therapy for ALS: A review. *Molecular Therapy: The Journal of the American Society of Gene Therapy* 29(12):3345–3358.

Andrew, A., J. Zhou, J. Gui, A. Harrison, X. Shi, M. Li, B. Guetti, R. Nathan, M. Tischbein, E. P. Pioro, E. Stommel, and W. Bradley. 2021. Pesticides applied to crops and amyotrophic lateral sclerosis risk in the U.S. *Neurotoxicology* 87:128–135.

ASHG (American Society of Human Genetics). 2008. *The Genetic Information Nondiscrimination Act (GINA)*. https://www.ashg.org/advocacy/gina (accessed April 5, 2024).

Baloh, R. H., J. P. Johnson, P. Avalos, P. Allred, S. Svendsen, G. Gowing, K. Roxas, A. Wu, B. Donahue, S. Osborne, G. Lawless, B. Shelley, K. Wheeler, C. Prina, D. Fine, T. Kendra-Romito, H. Stokes, V. Manoukian, A. Muthukumaran, L. Garcia, M. G. Bañuelos, M. Godoy, C. Bresee, H. Yu, D. Drazin, L. Ross, R. Naruse, H. Babu, E. A. Macklin, A. Vo, A. Elsayegh, W. Tourtellotte, M. Maya, M. Burford, F. Diaz, C. G. Patil, R. A. Lewis, and C. N. Svendsen. 2022. Transplantation of human neural progenitor cells secreting GDNF into the spinal cord of patients with ALS: A Phase 1/2a trial. *Nature Medicine* 28(9):1813–1822.

Beard, J. D., L. S. Engel, D. B. Richardson, M. D. Gammon, C. Baird, D. M. Umbach, K. D. Allen, C. L. Stanwyck, J. Keller, D. P. Sandler, S. Schmidt, and F. Kamel. 2017. Military service, deployments, and exposures in relation to amyotrophic lateral sclerosis survival. *PLOS One* 12(10):E0185751.

Bedlack, R. S., T. Vaughan, P. Wicks, J. Heywood, E. Sinani, R. Selsov, E. A. Macklin, D. Schoenfeld, M. Cudkowicz, and A. Sherman. 2016. How common are ALS plateaus and reversals? *Neurology* 86(9):808–812.

Benatar, M., and J. Wuu. 2012. Presymptomatic studies in ALS: Rationale, challenges, and approach. *Neurology* 79(16):1732–1739.

Benatar, M., C. Stanislaw, E. Reyes, S. Hussain, A. Cooley, M. C. Fernandez, D. D. Dauphin, S.-C. Michon, P. M. Andersen, and J. Wuu. 2016. Presymptomatic ALS genetic counseling and testing. *Neurology* 86(24):2295–2302.

Benatar, M., V. Granit, P. M. Andersen, A.-L. Grignon, C. McHutchison, S. Cosentino, A. Malaspina, and J. Wuu. 2022a. Mild motor impairment as prodromal state in amyotrophic lateral sclerosis: A new diagnostic entity. *Brain* 145(10):3500–3508.

Benatar, M., J. Wuu, P. M. Andersen, R. C. Bucelli, J. A. Andrews, M. Otto, N. A. Farahany, E. A. Harrington, W. Chen, A. A. Mitchell, T. Ferguson, S. Chew, L. Gedney, S. Oakley, J. Heo, S. Chary, L. Fanning, D. Graham, P. Sun, Y. Liu, J. Wong, and S. Fradette. 2022b. Design of a randomized, placebo-controlled, phase 3 trial of tofersen initiated in clinically presymptomatic SOD1 variant carriers: The Atlas Study. *Neurotherapeutics* 19(4):1248–1258.

Benatar, M., S. A. Goutman, K. A. Staats, E. L. Feldman, M. Weisskopf, E. Talbott, K. D. Dave, N. M. Thakur, and A. Al-Chalabi. 2023a. A roadmap to ALS prevention: Strategies and priorities. *J Neurol Neurosurg Psychiatry* 94(5):399–402.

Benatar, M., M. R. Turner, and J. Wuu. 2023b. Presymptomatic amyotrophic lateral sclerosis: from characterization to prevention. *Curr Opin Neurol* 36:360–364.

Biogen. 2022. *Biogen and Ionis announce topline Phase 1 study results of investigational drug in C9orf72 amyotrophic lateral sclerosis.* Cambridge, MA: Biogen.

Chia, R., A. Chiò, and B. J. Traynor. 2018. Novel genes associated with amyotrophic lateral sclerosis: Diagnostic and clinical implications. *Lancet Neurology* 17(1):94–102.

Chiò, A., L. Mazzini, S. D'alfonso, L. Corrado, A. Canosa, C. Moglia, U. Manera, E. Bersano, M. Brunetti, M. Barberis, J. H. Veldink, L. H. Van Den Berg, N. Pearce, W. Sproviero, R. Mclaughlin, A. Vajda, O. Hardiman, J. Rooney, G. Mora, A. Calvo, and A. Al-Chalabi. 2018. The multistep hypothesis of ALS revisited: The role of genetic mutations. *Neurology* 91(7):E635–E642.

Cui, C., J. Sun, K. A. Mckay, C. Ingre, and F. Fang. 2022. Medication use and risk of amyotrophic lateral sclerosis—A systematic review. *BMC Medicine* 20(1):251.

End the Legacy. 2023. *Genetic ALS and FTD pre-symptomatic population: FDA patient-led listening session.* https://www.endthelegacy.org/fda-listeneing-session (accessed April 5, 2024).

End the Legacy. 2024. *Presymptomatic/asymptomatic medical testing.* https://www.endthelegacy.org/presymptomatic-medical-testing (accessed May 16, 2024).

Evans, J. P., C. Skrzynia, and W. Burke. 2001. The complexities of predictive genetic testing. *BMJ* 322(7293):1052–1056.

Fang, T., G. Je, P. Pacut, K. Keyhanian, J. Gao, and M. Ghasemi. 2022. Gene therapy in amyotrophic lateral sclerosis. *Cells* 11(13):29.

Ferrari, R., D. Kapogiannis, E. D. Huey, and P. Momeni. 2011. FTD and ALS: A tale of two diseases. *Curr Alzheimer Res* 8(3):273–294.

Goutman, S. A., and E. L. Feldman. 2020. Voicing the need for amyotrophic lateral sclerosis environmental research. *JAMA Neurology* 77(5):543–544.

Goutman, S. A., J. Boss, C. Godwin, B. Mukherjee, E. L. Feldman, and S. A. Batterman. 2022a. Associations of self-reported occupational exposures and settings to ALS: A case-control study. *Int Arch Occup Environ Health* 95(7):1567–1586.

Goutman, S. A., J. Boss, C. Godwin, B. Mukherjee, E. L. Feldman, and S. A. Batterman. 2022b. Occupational history associates with ALS survival and onset segment. *Amyotroph Lateral Scler Frontotemporal Degener* 1–11.

Goutman, S. A., M. G. Savelieff, D. G. Jang, J. Hur, and E. L. Feldman. 2023. The amyotrophic lateral sclerosis exposome: Recent advances and future directions. *Nat Rev Neurol* 19(10):617–634.

Grzymski, J. J., G. Elhanan, J. A. Morales Rosado, E. Smith, K. A. Schlauch, R. Read, C. Rowan, N. Slotnick, S. Dabe, W. J. Metcalf, B. Lipp, H. Reed, L. Sharma, E. Levin, J. Kao, M. Rashkin, J. Bowes, K. Dunaway, A. Slonim, N. Washington, M. Ferber, A. Bolze, and J. T. Lu. 2020. Population genetic screening efficiently identifies carriers of autosomal dominant diseases. *Nature Medicine* 26(8):1235–1239.

Hanby, M. F., K. M. Scott, W. Scotton, L. Wijesekera, T. Mole, C. E. Ellis, P. Nigel Leigh, C. E. Shaw, and A. Al-Chalabi. 2011. The risk to relatives of patients with sporadic amyotrophic lateral sclerosis. *Brain* 134(12):3454–3457.

Harrison, D., P. Mehta, M. A. Van Es, E. Stommel, V. E. Drory, B. Nefussy, L. H. Van Den Berg, J. Crayle, and R. Bedlack. 2018. ALS reversals: Demographics, disease characteristics, treatments, and co-morbidities. *Amyotroph Lateral Scler Frontotemp Degener* 19(7–8):495–499.

IOM (Institute of Medicine). 2006. *Amyotrophic lateral sclerosis in veterans: Review of the scientific literature.* Washington, DC: The National Academies Press.

Klein, S. M., S. Behrstock, J. McHugh, K. Hoffmann, K. Wallace, M. Suzuki, P. Aebischer, and C. N. Svendsen. 2005. GDNF delivery using human neural progenitor cells in a rat model of ALS. *Hum Gene Ther* 16(4):509–521.

Klepek, H. N. 2018. *Genetic testing in amyotrophic lateral sclerosis: A survey of ALS clinicians and commercial testing laboratories.* Columbus, OH: The Ohio State University.

Korobeynikov, V. A., A. K. Lyashchenko, B. Blanco-Redondo, P. Jafar-Nejad, and N. A. Shneider. 2022. Antisense oligonucleotide silencing of FUS expression as a therapeutic approach in amyotrophic lateral sclerosis. *Nature Medicine* 28(1):104–116.

McKay, K. A., K. A. Smith, L. Smertinaite, F. Fang, C. Ingre, and F. Taube. 2021. Military service and related risk factors for amyotrophic lateral sclerosis. *Acta Neurol Scand* 143(1):39–50.

Mehta, P., J. Raymond, M. K. Han, T. Larson, J. D. Berry, S. Paganoni, H. Mitsumoto, R. S. Bedlack, and D. K. Horton. 2021. Recruitment of patients with amyotrophic lateral sclerosis for clinical trials and epidemiological studies: Descriptive study of the National ALS Registry's research notification mechanism. *J Med Internet Res* 23(12):E28021.

MGH (Massachusetts General Hospital). 2023. *Prevent ALS.* https://www.massgeneral.org/neurology/als/research/prevent-als (accessed June 10, 2024).

Mitsumoto, H., D. C. Garofalo, M. Gilmore, L. Andrews, R. M. Santella, H. Andrews, M. McElhiney, J. Murphy, J. W. Nieves, J. Rabkin, J. Hupf, D. K. Horton, P. Mehta, and P. Factor-Litvak. 2022. Case-control study in ALS using the National ALS Registry: Lead and agricultural chemicals are potential risk factors. *Amyotroph Lateral Scler Frontotempor Degener* 23(3–4):190–202.

Nazareth, S. B., G. A. Lazarin, and J. D. Goldberg. 2015. Changing trends in carrier screening for genetic disease in the United States. *Prenat Diagn* 35(10):931–935.

Newell, M. E., S. Adhikari, and R. U. Halden. 2022. Systematic and state-of the science review of the role of environmental factors in amyotrophic lateral sclerosis (ALS) or Lou Gehrig's disease. *Sci Total Environ* 817:152504.

Nguyen, H. P., C. Van Broeckhoven, and J. Van Der Zee. 2018. ALS genes in the genomic era and their implications for FTD. *Trends Genet* 34(6):404–423.

Oliveri, S., F. Ferrari, A. Manfrinati, and G. Pravettoni. 2018. A systematic review of the psychological implications of genetic testing: A comparative analysis among cardiovascular, neurodegenerative and cancer diseases. *Front Genet* 9:624.

Pfeiffer, R. M., B. Mayer, R. W. Kuncl, D. P. Check, E. K. Cahoon, D. R. Rivera, and D. M. Freedman. 2020. Identifying potential targets for prevention and treatment of amyotrophic lateral sclerosis based on a screen of Medicare prescription drugs. *Amyotroph Lateral Scler Frontotempor Degener* 21(3–4):235–245.

Ray, F. 2021. *Ionis opening Phase 3 trial of Ion363, antisense therapy for FUS-ALS.* https://alsnewstoday.com/news/ionis-opening-phase-3-trial-ion363-antisense-therapy-for-fus-als (accessed April 5, 2024).

Roberts, J. S., A. K. Patterson, and W. R. Uhlmann. 2020. Genetic testing for neurodegenerative diseases: Ethical and health communication challenges. *Neurobiol Dis* 141:104871.

Roggenbuck, J., B. H. F. Eubank, J. Wright, M. B. Harms, and S. J. Kolb. 2023. Evidence-based consensus guidelines for ALS genetic testing and counseling. *Ann Clin Transl Neurol* 10(11):2074–2091.

Ryan, M., M. Heverin, R. L. Mclaughlin, and O. Hardiman. 2019. Lifetime risk and heritability of amyotrophic lateral sclerosis. *JAMA Neurology* 76(11):1367–1374.

Suzuki, M., J. McHugh, C. Tork, B. Shelley, S. M. Klein, P. Aebischer, and C. N. Svendsen. 2007. GDNF secreting human neural progenitor cells protect dying motor neurons, but not their projection to muscle, in a rat model of familial ALS. *PLOS One* 2(8):E689.

Svendsen, C. N. 2023. *CNS10-NPC-GDNF delivered to the motor cortex for ALS.* https://clinicaltrials.gov/study/nct05306457 (accessed April 5, 2024).

University of Miami. 2024. *Guiding clinical care for people at risk for ALS and FTD.* https://news.med.miami.edu/guiding-clinical-care-for-people-at-risk-for-als-and-ftd (accessed May 14, 2024).

Vajda, A., R. L. McLaughlin, M. Heverin, O. Thorpe, S. Abrahams, A. Al-Chalabi, and O. Hardiman. 2017. Genetic testing in ALS: A survey of current practices. *Neurology* 88(10):991–999.

Van Rheenen, W., A. Shatunov, A. M. Dekker, R. L. McLaughlin, F. P. Diekstra, S. L. Pulit, R. A. Van Der Spek, et al. 2016. Genome-wide association analyses identify new risk variants and the genetic architecture of amyotrophic lateral sclerosis. *Nat Genet* 48(9): 1043–1048.

Vasta, R., R. Chia, B. J. Traynor, and A. Chiò. 2022. Unraveling the complex interplay between genes, environment, and climate in ALS. *EBioMedicine* 75:103795.

Vucic, S., H. J. Westeneng, A. Al-Chalabi, L. H. Van Den Berg, P. Talman, and M. C. Kiernan. 2019. Amyotrophic lateral sclerosis as a multi-step process: An Australia population study. *Amyotroph Lateral Scler Frontotemporal Degener* 20(7–8):532–537.

Vucic, S., M. Higashihara, G. Sobue, N. Atsuta, Y. Doi, S. Kuwabara, S. H. Kim, I. Kim, K. W. Oh, J. Park, E. M. Kim, P. Talman, P. Menon, and M. C. Kiernan. 2020. ALS is a multistep process in South Korean, Japanese, and Australian patients. *Neurology* 94(15):E1657–E1663.

Wagner, K. N., H. Nagaraja, D. C. Allain, A. Quick, S. Kolb, and J. Roggenbuck. 2017. Patients with amyotrophic lateral sclerosis have high interest in and limited access to genetic testing. *J Genet Couns* 26(3):604–611.

Wave Life Sciences USA. 2023. *Wave Life Sciences announces topline results from Phase 1b/2a Focus-C9 study of WVE-004 for C9orf72-associated amyotrophic lateral sclerosis and frontotemporal dementia.* Cambridge, MA: Wave Life Sciences USA.

Zhang, S., J. Cooper-Knock, A. K. Weimer, M. Shi, T. Moll, J. N. G. Marshall, C. Harvey, H. G. Nezhad, J. Franklin, C. D. S. Souza, K. Ning, C. Wang, J. Li, A. A. Dilliott, S. Farhan, E. Elhaik, I. Pasniceanu, M. R. Livesey, C. Eitan, E. Hornstein, K. P. Kenna, I. Blair, N. R. Wray, M. Kiernan, M. Mitne Neto, A. Chiò, R. Cauchi, W. Robberecht, P. Van Damme, P. Corcia, P. Couratier, O. Hardiman, R. Mclaughin, M. Gotkine, V. Drory, N. Ticozzi, V. Silani, J. H. Veldink, L. H. Van Den Berg, M. De Carvalho, J. S. Mora Pardina, M. Povedano, P. Andersen, M. Weber, N. A. Başak, A. Al-Chalabi, C. Shaw, P. J. Shaw, K. E. Morrison, J. E. Landers, J. D. Glass, J. H. Veldink, L. Ferraiuolo, P. J. Shaw, and M. P. Snyder. 2022. Genome-wide identification of the genetic basis of amyotrophic lateral sclerosis. *Neuron* 110(6):992–1008.

A

Public Session Agendas

First Committee Meeting
Public Session Agenda

Thursday, March 23, 2024
1:30 p.m.–3:00 p.m. (ET)
Virtual

OPEN SESSION

1:30 p.m.	**Welcome and Introductions** *ALAN I. LESHNER*, Committee Chair Chief Executive Officer, Emeritus American Association for the Advancement of Science
1:35 p.m.	**Presentation of the Charge to the Committee** *WALTER KOROSHETZ* Director, National Institute of Neurological Disorders and Stroke, National Institutes of Health
2:00 p.m.	**Discussion with Committee**
2:45 p.m.	**Public Comments**
3:00 p.m.	**Adjourn Open Session**

Second Committee Meeting
Public Session Agenda

Thursday, May 18, 2023
9:30 a.m.–12:00 p.m. (ET)
Hybrid

OPEN SESSION

9:30 a.m.	**Welcome and Opening Remarks** *ALAN I. LESHNER*, Committee Chair Chief Executive Officer, Emeritus American Association for the Advancement of Science

SESSION 1   WHAT TOOLS DO ALS NONPROFITS NEED TO BE MORE EFFECTIVE AND IMPACTFUL?

9:40 a.m.	**Panel Session Remarks** *Virtual Participants*

- Dan Doctoroff, Target ALS
- Sunny Brous, Her ALS Story
- Juliet Pierce, Paralyzed Veterans of America
- Indu Navar, Everything ALS
- Penny Dacks, Association for Frontotemporal Degeneration
- Jean Swidler, Genetic ALS & FTD: End the Legacy
- Blair Casey, Team Gleason
- Jinsy Andrews and James Berry, Northeast ALS (NEALS) Consortium
- Benzi Kluger, International Neuropalliative Care Society

10:20 a.m.	**Break**
10:30 a.m.	**Panel Session Remarks** *In-Person Participants*

- Neil Thakur, ALS Association
- Cathy Collet, More Than Our Stories
- Sonya Elling, I AM ALS
- Paul Melmeyer, Muscular Dystrophy Association

11:15 a.m.	**Discussion with Committee**
12:00 p.m.	**Adjourn Open Session**

Public Workshop
Public Session Agenda

Thursday, August 10, 2023
12:00 p.m.–3:10 p.m. (ET)
Virtual

OPEN SESSION

12:00 p.m.   **Welcome and Opening Remarks**
              JOSHUA M. SHARFSTEIN, Committee Member
              Vice Dean for Public Health Practice and Community
              Engagement, Johns Hopkins Bloomberg School of Public
              Health

SESSION 1   PANEL ON INSURANCE COVERAGE FOR ALS CARE

12:05 p.m.   Medicare and Medicaid
              TERRI POSTMA
              Senior Medical Officer, Centers for Medicare & Medicaid
              Services

              Home Health Care for Veterans Living with ALS
              RENEE GOLDEN
              Regional Director, Military & Federal Homecare, Maxim
              Healthcare Services

              Private Insurance
              LISA M. LATTS
              Senior Medical Director, Value Based Care, Optum Health
              Medical Office

12:35 p.m.   **Discussion with Committee**

1:00 p.m.   **Break**

SESSION 2   PANEL ON NAVIGATING ALS CARE AND PAYMENT

1:10 p.m.   Lived Experience Perspective
                BRUCE ROSENBLUM
                Vice President of Content and Workflow Solutions, Wiley
                Person Living with ALS

                Navigating ALS Care and Payment with People Living with
                ALS
                COLLEEN HOARTY
                Medical Social Worker
                University of Nebraska Medical Center

                MELANIE LENDNAL
                Senior Vice President, Policy and Advocacy, ALS
                Association

                JOANNE LYNN
                Eldercare Consultant

1:50 p.m.   **Discussion with Committee**

SESSION 3   PERSPECTIVES ON NEEDS AND OPPORTUNITIES IN THE ALS MULTIDISCIPLINARY CARE MODEL

2:05 p.m.   ALS Multidisciplinary Care Model—ALS Association
                Certification
                LORI BANKER-HORNER
                Senior Director, Clinical Programs, ALS Association

                ALS Multidisciplinary Care Model—MDA Certification
                NORA CAPOCCI
                Vice President, Healthcare Services
                Chief Privacy Officer, Muscular Dystrophy Association

2:25 p.m.   **Discussion with Committee**

SESSION 4   ALS Multidisciplinary Care-Provider Perspectives

2:05 p.m.   Provider Perspectives
TERRY HEIMAN-PATTERSON,
Director, MDA/ALS Center of Hope,
Temple University

JOHN HANSEN-FLASCHEN,
Founding Medical Director, Paul Harron Lung Center
University of Pennsylvania

2:55 p.m.   **Discussion with Committee**

3:10 p.m.   **Adjourn Open Session**

**Public Workshop
Public Session Agenda**

**Wednesday, August 23, 2023
12:00 p.m.–3:00 p.m. (ET)
Virtual**

OPEN SESSION

9:30 a.m.   **Welcome and Opening Remarks**
ALAN I. LESHNER, Committee Chair
Chief Executive Officer, Emeritus, American Association for
the Advancement of Science

SESSION 1   UNDERSTANDING LIVING WITH ALS

Sarah Lunsford, Moderator

12:15 p.m.   **Panel Session Remarks**
- Desi Kessler, person living with ALS
- Paul Siefert, person living with ALS
- Asia Jami, person living with ALS
- Jim and Sylvia Clingman, person living with ALS and caregiver

SESSION 2   THE COST OF CARE

Sarah Lunsford, Moderator

1:00 p.m.   **Panel Session Remarks**
  - Ron Faretra, person living with ALS
  - Kristin Rankin, person living with ALS
  - Julian Rodriguez, person living with ALS
  - Jean Swidler, presymptomatic genetic carrier and caregiver

1:45 p.m.   **Break**

SESSION 3   EXPLORING THE CAREGIVER EXPERIENCE

Sarah Lunsford, Moderator

2:00 p.m.   **Panel Session Remarks**
  - Katrina Byrd, Caregiver
  - Vanessa Jackson, Caregiver
  - Siobhan Pandya, Caregiver
  - Ashley Lee, Caregiver

2:45 p.m.   **Closing Remarks**

3:00 p.m.   **Adjourn Open Session**

Public Workshop
Public Session Agenda

Friday, September 1, 2023
12:00 p.m.–3:45 p.m. (ET)
Virtual

OPEN SESSION

12:00 p.m.   **Welcome and Opening Remarks**
ALAN I. LESHNER, Committee Chair
Chief Executive Officer, Emeritus, American Association for the Advancement of Science

SESSION 1   MEDICARE COVERAGE CHALLENGES IN ALS

Sarah Lunsford, Moderator

12:05 p.m.   *KATHLEEN HOLT*
Associate Director/Attorney, Center for Medicare Advocacy

SESSION 2   ALS EPIDEMIOLOGY AND RESEARCH

12:30 p.m.   *PAUL MEHTA*
Principal Investigator, National ALS Registry

SARAH FONTAINE
Program Manager, Congressionally Directed Medical
Research Programs, ALS Research Program, U.S.
Department of Defense

1:05 p.m.   **Break**

SESSION 3   ALS DRUG DEVELOPMENT

Academic Research and the ALS Drug Development Pipeline

1:50 p.m.   *JUSTIN ICHIDA*
Professor of Stem Cell Biology and Regenerative Medicine,
University of Southern California

FDA and NIH Public–Private Partnership—Critical Path for
Rare Neurodegenerative Disease (CP-RND)

COLLIN HOVINGA
Vice President, Rare and Orphan Disease Programs,
Critical Path Institute

ALS Therapy Development Institute (TDI)
FERNANDO VIEIRA
Chief Executive Officer and Chief Scientific Officer, ALS
Therapy Development Institute

Panel Session Remarks
- Michael Benatar, Professor of Neurology and Executive
  Director, the ALS Center, University of Miami
- Neil Thakur, Chief Mission Officer, ALS Association

SESSION 4   DESIGNING CLINICAL TRIALS IN ALS

2:35 p.m.   *JAMES BERRY*
               Director, Neurological Clinical Research Institute,
               Massachusetts General Hospital

               BOB HEBRON
               Chair, Clinical Trials Team, I AM ALS

3:05 p.m.   **Break**

**SESSION 5   PANEL ON LESSONS LEARNED FROM OTHER
               DISEASE AREAS**

               Lessons Learned—The Evolution of Cystic Fibrosis Care
3:10 p.m.   *ALBERT FARO*
               Vice President, Clinical Affairs, Cystic Fibrosis Foundation

               Patient-Reported Outcomes and Preferences

               NORAH CROSSNOHERE
               Assistant Professor, General Internal Medicine, Ohio State
               University College of Medicine

               Integrating Research and Clinical Care—Pediatric Oncology
               WILLIAM WOODS
               Professor Emeritus, Department of Pediatrics, Emory
               University School of Medicine

3:45 p.m.   **Closing Remarks**
3:45 p.m.   **Adjourn Open Session**

B

Biographical Sketches of Committee Members and Staff

COMMITTEE MEMBERS

Alan I. Leshner (*Chair*) is Chief Executive Officer, Emeritus, of the American Association for the Advancement of Science (AAAS) and former Executive Publisher of the journal *Science*. Before joining AAAS, Dr. Leshner was Director of the National Institute on Drug Abuse at the National Institutes of Health. He also served as Deputy Director and Acting Director of the National Institute of Mental Health, and in several roles at the National Science Foundation. Previously, Dr. Leshner was Professor of Psychology at Bucknell University. Dr. Leshner is an elected fellow of AAAS, the American Academy of Arts and Sciences, and many others. He is a member and served as Vice Chair of the governing Council of the National Academy of Medicine of the National Academies of Sciences, Engineering, and Medicine. He served two terms on the National Science Board, appointed first by President Bush and then reappointed by President Obama. Dr. Leshner received M.S. and Ph.D. in physiological psychology from Rutgers University and an A.B. in psychology from Franklin and Marshall College. Dr. Leshner has received many honors and awards, including the Walsh McDermott Medal from the National Academy of Medicine and seven honorary Doctor of Science degrees.

Suma Babu is Assistant Professor of neurology at Harvard Medical School and co-director of the Neurological Clinical Research Institute at Massachusetts General Hospital (MGH) and provides clinical care for people with ALS and other motor neuron diseases at the multidisciplinary ALS

193

clinic at the MGH Sean M Healey and AMG Center for ALS. She has a special interest in developing disease modifying treatments and clinical trial biomarker readouts for people with motor neuron diseases. Her clinical research work is primarily aimed at improving ALS patient care and survival outcomes. As the overall principal investigator (PI), she has led two multisite, early-phase, biomarker-driven clinical trials in ALS (MN-166 in ALS-investigator initiated, LAM-002A in C9orf72 ALS-protocol PI for OrphAI therapeutics industry-sponsored trial). She serves as a multiple PI on several NIH-U01 expanded access protocols (EAPs), including the awarded Trehalose 25-site EAP (Seelos), Pridopidine 45 site EAP (Prilenia), and 10-site Autologus Treg infusion EAP (Rapa) funded under the Accelerating Access to Critical Therapies for ALS Act (ACT for ALS). As the MGH site PI, she leads Phase 1, 2, and 3 clinical trials evaluating novel therapeutics for genetic ALS. Dr. Babu serves on the MGH Healey Center Coordinating Center design and operations committee and serves as regimen co-lead for Regimens B and G (Biohaven and Denali) of the Healey ALS platform trial. She serves as faculty of the MGH clinical coordinating center for the gene therapy consortium for gene-based clinical trials conducted within the National Institute of Neurological Diseases and Stroke (NINDS) NeuroNEXT network. As of March 2024, she serves as a compensated consultant for uniQure, a gene therapy company. Dr. Babu has also previously consulted with Medscape and served on a Biogen advisory board. Dr. Babu co-chairs the Northeast Amyotrophic Lateral Sclerosis (NEALS) Consortium imaging subcommittee, an international organization for ALS researchers. Her research is funded by awards from NINDS of the National Institutes of Health (NIH). Dr. Babu is one of the multiple PIs leading the Access for All in ALS East Clinical Coordinating Center awarded by NINDS to MGH funded under the ACT for ALS. Dr. Babu completed her neurology training at the Cleveland Clinic, Ohio, and two fellowships in neuromuscular medicine and neurodegenerative disorders at Harvard Medical School. Her clinical research training includes the completion of a 2-year competitive Clinical and Translational Research Academy program at Harvard Medical School (2018), M.P.H. at the University of Maryland School of Public Health (2008), and a 1-year competitive NIH-funded Clinical Trial Methodology Course (2017 cohort).

Chelsey R. Carter is Assistant Professor of public health in the Department of Social and Behavioral Sciences at Yale School of Public Health. Dr. Carter has expertise in medicine, public health, and race. Her research program examines how scientific knowledge production, clinical care, and systemic marginalization impact historically underrepresented communities affected by neurodegenerative diseases, like ALS, and genomic medicine. Dr. Carter is also undertaking a book project that includes an ethnographic study of the diverse experiences of living with ALS, which draws on more than 15 years of experience with Black communities affected by ALS. Her scholarship has been funded by the National Science Foundation, the Andrew Mellon Foundation, the Wenner Gren Foundation, the Ford Foundation, the ALS Association, the National Institutes of Health, and more. She serves as an executive board member for the Society for Medical Anthropology, and from April 2022 to January 2023, Dr. Carter was a working group member for the National Institutes of Health/National Institute of Neurological Disorders and Stroke Strategic Plan on ALS. Dr. Carter has provided consulting services or made presentations to pharmaceutical companies and nonprofit organizations on issues of race, equity, and inclusion since 2020. Dr. Carter serves on the Care Services Committee for the ALS Association. Dr. Carter was a Presidential Postdoctoral Research Fellow at Princeton University in the Department of Anthropology and Center for Transnational Policing. She received her bachelor's degree in anthropology with a minor in Spanish (high honors) from Emory University. She holds a Ph.D. in sociocultural anthropology, an M.P.H., and a certificate in women, gender, and sexuality studies from Washington University in St. Louis.

Maceo Carter is 47 years old and was diagnosed with ALS 8 years ago on November 8, 2016. Two things he has learned during this ALS journey are (1) each person's journey is their own roller coaster filled with highs and lows, and (2) with the right amount of help it is amazing the life you can live, albeit with a terminal disease. Maceo believes all things happen for a reason and that he has been given the opportunity to help with something that seems insurmountable. He wants to change the outlook on ALS, the approach to caring for those living with ALS, and help people live the best life possible with this disease. Maceo works with the ALS Association and the Many Shades of ALS Team at I AM ALS. He is the father of four sons ages 24, 15, 13, and 2. He is still employed and works 40 hours per week. Before diagnosis, Maceo thoroughly enjoyed cooking, especially with his sons. He is a huge University of North Carolina basketball fan. He and his wife have known each other for more than 20 years and have been married for 9.

George Demiris is Penn Integrates Knowledge University Professor in the School of Nursing with a joint appointment in the Department of Biostatistics, Epidemiology, and Informatics in the Perelman School of Medicine, University of Pennsylvania. His research explores innovative ways to use inclusive technology and support patients and their families in various settings including homes and communities. He has conducted clinical trials to examine telehealth-based interventions for family caregivers in hospice. He also studies "smart home" solutions and digitally augmented residential settings to facilitate passive monitoring via telehealth, and support quality of life for older adults and people with disabilities. He is a member of the National Academy of Medicine and a Fellow of the Gerontological Society of America and the American College of Medical Informatics. He served on the National Academies' committee for the report *Health and Medical Dimensions of Social Isolation and Loneliness in Older Adults* (2020) and a National Academy of Medicine 2018 work group on technologies to enhance person, family, and community activation. He has presented his research at a National Academies' Forum on Aging, Disability, and Independence Workshop on the Role of Human Factors in Home Health Care and served as reviewer for the National Academies' report *The Promise of Assistive Technology to Enhance Activity and Work Participation* (2017).

John Dunlop is Chief Scientific Officer, Aliada Therapeutics, a central nervous system–focused drug development company advancing a differentiated approach for blood–brain barrier delivery of a range of biologic therapeutics. Until August 2023, he was head of research and development at Neumora, a company launched to pursue an innovative approach to precision medicines for brain diseases. Prior to Neumora, Dr. Dunlop was at Amgen, where he led the neuroscience research program responsible for therapeutic discovery activities in neurodegenerative diseases, pain, and migraine. Prior to Amgen, he led neuroscience discovery and early development at AstraZeneca and previously held executive leadership roles in neuroscience at Wyeth and Pfizer. Dr. Dunlop is an industry member of the HEAL (Helping End Addiction Long term) Partnership Committee, a National Institutes of Health (NIH) advisory committee established to support NIH initiatives launched to address the nation's opioid crisis. He is a board member of Target-ALS, a nonprofit enterprise dedicated to accelerating drug discovery and development in ALS, and the Massachusetts Biotechnology Council (MassBio), and he is on the scientific advisory boards of Vigil Neuroscience and the Packard Center for ALS Research at Johns Hopkins. Dr. Dunlop holds a B.Sc. in biochemistry from the University of Glasgow and a Ph.D. in neuroscience from the University of St. Andrews.

Eva L. Feldman is James W. Albers Distinguished University Professor, Russell N. DeJong Professor of Neurology, and Director of the ALS Center of Excellence at the University of Michigan (ALS Centers of Excellence receive some funding from the ALS Association to support patient care). With 30 years of continuous funding from the National Institutes of Health, she was the principal investigator on the first two U.S. Food and Drug Administration–approved stem cell transplant clinical trials for ALS. Related to her work in stem cell transplant treatments for ALS, Dr. Feldman previously worked with biotech companies (e.g., NeuroStem Inc. and Seneca) on the clinical translation of her research. Dr. Feldman also had a one-time consulting relationship with Biogen in 2022 regarding ALS therapies. Feldman recently received a National Institutes of Health Director's Transformative Award for her groundbreaking research on the ALS exposome, as well as separate grants from the National Institute of Environmental Health Sciences and the Centers for Disease Control and Prevention for her work on linking environmental pollutants with ALS, and the National Institute of Neurological Disorders and Stroke (NINDS) on how immunity contributes to ALS risk. Since December 2023, she has been a participant in the Neural Exposome Strategic Plan Working Group being convened by the NINDS Office of Neural Exposome & Toxicology to consider high-impact exposomic research opportunities. Dr. Feldman is an author of the 2022 Lancet ALS seminar outlining the current state of ALS diagnosis, clinical care, and research. At the University of Michigan, she directs a research program of 25 scientists and has more than 500 publications. Dr. Feldman served as President of the American Neurological Association (2011–2013), the third woman to hold this position in 130 years, and she has received lifetime achievement awards from multiple societies. She is an elected member of the National Academy of Medicine. Dr. Feldman received her M.D. and Ph.D. from the University of Michigan, completed neurology residency at Johns Hopkins, and a neuromuscular fellowship at the University of Michigan.

Holly Fernandez Lynch is Assistant Professor of medical ethics and law at the University of Pennsylvania. She pursues conceptual and empirical scholarship regarding clinical research ethics and regulation, access to investigational medicines outside clinical trials, and U.S. Food and Drug Administration pharmaceutical policy, especially early approval pathways for diseases with unmet treatment needs. She is a board member of Public Responsibility in Medicine & Research and the American Society for Law, Medicine, and Ethics, as well as a fellow of the Hastings Center and a National Academy of Medicine Emerging Leader in Health and Medicine. She served as Ethicist in Residence at the Robert Wood Johnson Foundation from 2020 to 2023, and, as of January 2024, serves on the Observational Study Monitoring Board for the new Access for All in ALS consortium. She has previously worked as an attorney in private practice, a bioethicist serving the National Institutes of Health's Division of AIDS, an analyst with President Obama's Commission for the Study of Bioethical Issues, and Executive Director of Harvard Law School's bioethics and health law research program. She earned graduate degrees in law and bioethics at the University of Pennsylvania.

Ileana Howard is a physical medicine and rehabilitation physician specializing in the care of persons with ALS. She currently serves as Chair of the ALS Executive Committee for the Veterans Health Administration as well as caring for patients and families as the Medical Co-Director of the

ALS Center of Excellence at the VA Puget Sound in Seattle, Washington. Dr. Howard is Associate Professor of rehabilitation medicine at the University of Washington. She has volunteered for the board of the American Association of Neuromuscular and Electrodiagnostic Medicine (AANEM) and the ALS Association Evergreen Chapter. She was awarded the Clinical Excellence Award by the Paralyzed Veterans of America (PVA) in 2018, and the Advocacy Award by the AANEM in 2021. She has previously received honorarium for her work with AANEM, PVA, and for consulting on a PBS film on individuals living with ALS. Dr. Howard also serves on the national Medical Advisory Board and local Evergreen Chapter Leadership Council for the ALS Association. Dr. Howard is currently providing her expertise as part of an AANEM effort to develop expert-based consensus guidelines for an ALS home health and durable medical equipment medical standard. She has numerous publications and national presentations on the rehabilitation management of ALS. Dr. Howard received her undergraduate degree at Smith College and received a Fulbright fellowship to study public health in Spain prior to completing her medical doctorate at Harvard Medical School. She completed an internal medicine internship at the Lahey Clinic, followed by a physical medicine and rehabilitation residency at the University of Washington. She maintains dual board certifications in physical medicine and rehabilitation and electrodiagnostic medicine.

Jerome E. Kurent is Professor of neurology and medicine at the Medical University of South Carolina and Director of the ALS Interdisciplinary Clinic at the Ralph H. Johnson Veterans Affairs Medical Center in Charleston, South Carolina. His primary research and educational outreach have focused on palliative and end-of-life care for patients with incurable neurological diseases including ALS, as well as public policy related to providing care for persons with ALS. His research has also included a focus on improving quality of life for African American patients with incurable end-stage diseases. Dr. Kurent is co-editor of *Public Policy in ALS/MND Care: An International Perspective* and *A Clinician's Guide to Palliative Care*. He served as a member of the National Hospice and Palliative Care Organization ALS Work Group. His honors and awards include the Lifetime Achievement Award from the International Neuropalliative Care Society (2021); Faculty Scholar of the Project on Death in America; and Fellow, Mayday Pain and Society. Dr. Kurent received his M.D. from the University of Cincinnati, M.S. from The Ohio State University, and M.P.H. from the Harvard T.H. Chan School of Public Health. He completed residencies in neurology and internal medicine at the Johns Hopkins Hospital. He completed fellowships in neurovirology, neuromuscular diseases, and electromyography at the National Institutes of Health and in geriatric medicine from Harvard.

Won Young Lee is Associate Professor in the Division of Pulmonary and Critical Care Medicine at the University of Texas Southwestern Medical Center in Dallas. Dr. Lee serves as Medical Director of the Clinical Center for Sleep and Breathing Disorders Center and has worked at UT Southwestern for 15 years as an academic faculty, in the clinician educator track. Dr. Lee is board certified in internal medicine, pulmonary medicine, critical care medicine, and sleep medicine. Dr. Lee brings pulmonary expertise in managing patients with chronic respiratory failure relevant to neuromuscular conditions, including ALS, muscular dystrophy, postpolio syndrome, spinal cord injury, diaphragm disorders, myasthenia gravis, and inflammatory muscle or neurologic conditions. In addition, he has expertise in sleep medicine, and continues to practice both pulmonary and critical care medicine. Dr. Lee has received numerous teaching awards, including, most recently, the Regents Outstanding Teaching Award for the State of Texas in 2019. Dr. Lee received his M.D. from the University of Nevada, Reno, School of Medicine and completed internal medicine residency at University of Nevada Affiliated Hospitals. Dr. Lee completed a Pulmonary and Critical Care Fellowship at Rush University Medical Center, Chicago, and a Sleep Medicine Fellowship at the University of Chicago.

Harold L. Paz is an operating partner at Khosla Ventures focused on health care and life science companies. Previously, Dr. Paz was Professor of medicine at the Renaissance School of Medicine, Stony Brook University, where he was also Executive Vice President for Health Sciences and Chief Executive Officer of Stony Brook University Medicine. Dr. Paz has also served as Executive Vice President and Chancellor for health affairs at The Ohio State University (OSU) and Chief Executive Officer of the Ohio State Wexner Medical Center. Before joining OSU, Dr. Paz was Executive Vice President and Chief Medical Officer at CVS Health/Aetna, where he led clinical strategy and policy for Aetna's domestic and global businesses. He has served on numerous health care and biotechnology boards and is currently a member of the National Academy of Medicine Leadership Consortium, the board of directors of Research!America and Envision Health, and the medical advisory board of Curai Health. Dr. Paz previously served on the Board of Directors for Select Medical, which provides rehabilitation and postacute care services, and United Surgical Partners International, an ambulatory surgery company. Dr. Paz received his bachelor's degree from the University of Rochester, a master's degree in life science engineering from Tufts University, and his M.D. from the University of Rochester. He completed his residency at Northwestern University. Dr. Paz was a Eudowood Fellow in pulmonary and critical care at the Johns Hopkins Medical School and a postdoctoral fellow in environmental health science at the Johns Hopkins School of Hygiene and Public Health.

Tonya J. Roberts is Associate Professor and Karen Frick Pridham Professor in Family-Centered Care in the School of Nursing at the University of Wisconsin–Madison. Dr. Roberts's research is focused on optimizing person- and family-centered care to improve quality of life for vulnerable older adults who require long-term care, with a particular emphasis on promoting autonomy, dignity, and meaningful living in nursing homes. Her research focuses on identifying ways to increase patient and family engagement in care planning and aligning care with patient and family preferences, priorities, and goals. She has prior experience in direct care, nursing, and nursing leadership roles in long-term care settings. She is Affiliate of the Center for Aging Research and Education at the University of Wisconsin and a member of Advancing Excellence, the Moving Forward Coalition, and the Gerontological Society of America. Dr. Roberts received a B.S., M.S., and Ph.D. from the University of Wisconsin–Madison and completed a postdoctoral fellowship with the U.S. Department of Veterans Affairs. She has formal training in nursing, industrial and systems engineering, and health services research.

Rita Sattler is Professor of translational neuroscience at the Barrow Neurological Institute in Phoenix, Arizona. Her research is focused on mechanisms of neurodegeneration in varying dementias, including frontotemporal dementia (FTD), FTD with motor neuron dysfunction (FTD/ALS), Alzheimer's disease, and Lewy Body dementia using human model systems, including postmortem autopsy tissues and human patient-derived induced pluripotent stem cells differentiated into neurons and glial cells. Dr. Sattler is a member of the American Society for Neuroscience and the American Society for Neurochemistry. She is the recipient of several awards and fellowships, including the Governor's Gold Medal for the highest academic achievement in graduate studies at the University of Toronto and a Human Frontier Science Program Long-term Fellowship. Dr. Sattler serves in uncompensated advisory roles for the Robert Packard Center for ALS Research, Milken Foundation, LiveLikeLou Foundation, Spinogenix Inc., and Korro Bio Inc. Dr. Sattler serves on the Scientific Advisory Boards of the Northeast Amyotrophic Lateral Sclerosis (NEALS) Consortium and a new scientific program on FTD sponsored by the Milken Institute and the Kissick Family Foundation. In addition, Dr. Sattler has worked with Regenesis Biomedical Inc. Dr. Sattler received her master's and doctorate degrees from the University of Toronto and performed her postdoctoral training in the Department of Neuroscience at Johns Hopkins University. She then served as lead scientist for a small startup company overseeing assay development and drug screening of lead compounds for ALS, in addition to the validation of disease biomarkers. From there, Dr. Sattler joined the Drug Discovery Center at Johns Hopkins University to strengthen her expertise in preclinical drug development. She started her first faculty position as Assistant Professor of neurology in 2012 at Johns Hopkins University.

Joel Shamaskin is Professor Emeritus of medicine (retired) at the University of Rochester School of Medicine and Dentistry. He served as Chief Resident in Primary Care Internal Medicine, Fellow in Geriatric Medicine, Attending Physician at Strong Memorial Hospital, and Site Medical Director in the University of Rochester Primary Care Network. He was a clinical educator and practiced primary care internal medicine for 31 years until his ALS diagnosis in 2016. Since 2017 he has been actively involved in various ALS advocacy efforts. Dr. Shamaskin has previously received honorarium from the ALS Association and the Institute for Clinical and Economic Review related to his work in ALS. He was elected a Fellow of the American College of Physicians in 1996 and was the recipient of the James M. Stewart Outstanding Teaching award from the University of Rochester in 2014. He received his M.D. at the University of Virginia in 1980 and completed residency training at the University of Rochester School of Medicine and Dentistry.

Joshua Sharfstein is Vice Dean for public health practice and community engagement and Professor of the practice in health policy and management at the Johns Hopkins Bloomberg School of Public Health. He formerly served as Principal Deputy Commissioner of the U.S. Food and Drug Administration and Secretary of Maryland's Department of Health and Mental Hygiene. He is an elected member of the National Academy of Medicine and Fellow of the National Academy of Public Administration. A board certified pediatrician, he graduated from Harvard Medical School in 1996, the Boston Combined Residency Program in Pediatrics in 1999, and the fellowship in General Academic Pediatrics at the Boston University School of Medicine in 2001. Dr. Sharfstein is working on a part-time federal detail to the National Institutes of Health to support efforts to develop a national hepatitis C elimination effort.

Anantha Shekhar is Senior Vice-Chancellor for the health sciences and John and Gertrude Petersen Dean of the School of Medicine at the University of Pittsburgh. He is a nationally recognized educator, researcher, and entrepreneur with major contributions in medicine and life sciences. At Pitt, Dr. Shekhar leads all six health sciences schools that, for more than a century, have led education and research in their respective fields, propelling scientific discovery and clinical innovation that advance human health. Education at the Schools of the Health Sciences—dental medicine, health and rehabilitation sciences, medicine, nursing, pharmacy, and public health—emphasizes individualized curricula and interprofessional team-based instruction to train students in core competencies of their chosen health professions while also preparing them as advocates, innovators, and stewards of responsible, inclusive health care delivery. Innovation, transformation, and successful collaborations across the private, public, and philanthropic sectors have defined Dr. Shekhar's career. His areas of expertise include basic and clinical research on neuropsychiatric disorders and clinical neuropharmacology. His laboratory has developed several translational models for neuropsychiatric disorders as well as identified novel targets for neuropsychiatric disorder treatments in commercial development. Grants from the National Institutes of Health, private foundations, and commercial collaborations have supported his research. He has co-authored more than 200 original scientific papers published in leading basic science and clinical journals. He is a founder of multiple biotech companies developing novel therapies. Dr. Shekhar is a member of the National Academies of Sciences, Engineering, and Medicine's Forum on Drug Discovery, Development, and Translation. Dr. Shekhar, who was born in India, earned his M.D. at St. John's Medical College, Bangalore, and Ph.D. in neuroscience at Indiana University.

Mindy Uhrlaub is an author and familial ALS activist. She is a presymptomatic carrier of the fatal gene C9orf72, which causes ALS and frontotemporal dementia (FTD). She has won several awards for her writing, including the 2021 NYC Big Book Award for Cultural Heritage. For the writing of her forthcoming book, *A War of Nerves: An ALS Memoir*, she has been awarded residencies at Millay Arts, the Hambidge Center, and Joyce Maynard's Write by the Lake. She is participating in more than a dozen longitudinal studies of ALS/FTD and, through ALS & FTD: End the Legacy, an organization that advocates for carriers of genetic ALS, has testified before the U.S. Food and Drug Administration in an opening listening session about the needs of premanifest carriers of ALS genes.

NATIONAL ACADEMIES STAFF

Rebecca A. English (*Study Director*) is Senior Program Officer in the Board on Health Sciences Policy at the National Academies of Sciences, Engineering, and Medicine. She has directed, co-directed, and staffed a number of projects at the National Academies including, most recently, the Forum on Temporomandibular Disorders (2023-present), Realizing the Promise of Equity in the Organ Transplantation System (2022), Assessment of Strategies for Managing Cancer Risks Associated with Radiation Exposure During Crewed Space Missions (2021), and Necessity, Use, and Care of Laboratory Dogs at the U.S. Department of Veterans Affairs (2020). She staffed the Forum on Drug Discovery, Development, and Translation at the National Academies in various capacities between 2009 and 2016, working on wide-ranging projects related to the U.S. clinical trials enterprise as well as multidrug-resistant tuberculosis throughout the world. Prior to joining the National Academies, she worked on health policy for Congressman

Porter J. Goss (FL-14) and for the National Active and Retired Federal Employees Association. She holds an M.P.H. from the University of Michigan and a B.A. from the University of Notre Dame in political science.

Ashley Bologna is Senior Program Assistant in the Health Medicine Division at the National Academies of Sciences, Engineering, and Medicine. In addition to this study, she works on projects initiated by the Committee on Personal Protective Equipment for Workplace Safety and Health. This is a standing committee at the National Academies sponsored by the National Personal Protective Technology Laboratory of the National Institute for Occupational Safety and Health, to provide a forum for discussion of scientific and technical issues relevant to the development, certification, deployment, and use of personal protective equipment, standards, and related systems to ensure workplace safety and health. She earned her M.S. in global health at Georgetown University. She also has a B.A. in international relations and political science from Virginia Wesleyan University.

Lyle Carrera is Research Associate for the Board on Health Care Services at the National Academies of Sciences, Engineering, and Medicine. He has provided research support for several workshops and consensus studies, most recently including Sustaining Essential Health Care Services Related to Intimate Partner Violence During Public Health Emergencies and Study and Recommendations on the HIMS, FADAP, and Other Drug and Alcohol Programs within the USDOT. Before joining the National Academies, Carrera worked on equity assessment for Baltimore City's Bureau of the Budget and Management Research, as well as transportation safety policy research at the University of Nevada, Las Vegas. Carrera holds an M.S.P.H. in health policy from the Johns Hopkins Bloomberg School of Public Health and a B.A. in public health studies and political science from the Johns Hopkins University.

Sharyl Nass serves as Senior Director of the Board on Health Care Services and Director of the National Cancer Policy Forum at the National Academies of Sciences, Engineering, and Medicine. The National Academies provide independent, objective analysis and advice to the nation to solve complex problems and inform public policy decisions related to science, technology, and medicine. To enable the best possible care for all patients, the Board undertakes scholarly analysis of the organization, financing, effectiveness, workforce, and delivery of health care, with emphasis on quality, cost, and accessibility. The Cancer Forum examines policy issues pertaining to the entire continuum of cancer research and care. For more than two decades, Dr. Nass has worked on a broad range of health and science policy topics that includes the quality and safety of health care and clinical trials, developing technologies for precision medicine, and strategies for large-scale biomedical science. She has a Ph.D. in cell biology from Georgetown University and undertook postdoctoral training at the Johns Hopkins University School of Medicine, as well as a research fellowship at the Max Planck Institute in Germany. She also holds a B.S. and an M.S. from the University of Wisconsin–Madison. She has been the recipient of the Cecil Medal for Excellence in Health Policy Research, a Distinguished Service Award from the National Academies, and the Institute of Medicine staff team achievement award as team leader.

Clare Stroud is Senior Board Director for the Board on Health Sciences Policy at the National Academies of Sciences, Engineering, and Medicine. In this capacity, she oversees a program of activities aimed at fostering the basic biomedical and clinical research enterprises; addressing the ethical, legal, and social contexts of scientific and technologic advances related to health; and strengthening the preparedness, resilience, and sustainability of communities. Previously, she served as Director of the National Academies' Forum on Neuroscience and Nervous System Disorders, which brings together leaders from government, academia, industry, and nonprofit organizations to discuss key challenges and emerging issues in neuroscience research, development of therapies for nervous system disorders, and related ethical and societal issues. She also led consensus studies and contributed to projects on topics such as pain management, medications for opioid use disorder, traumatic brain injury, preventing cognitive decline and dementia, supporting persons living with dementia and their caregivers, the health and well-being of young adults, and disaster preparedness and response. Dr. Stroud first joined the National Academies as a Mirzayan Science and Technology Policy Graduate Fellow. She has also been an Associate at AmericaSpeaks, a nonprofit organization that engaged citizens in decision making on important public policy issues. Dr. Stroud received her Ph.D. from the University of Maryland, College Park, with research focused on the cognitive neuroscience of language, and her bachelor's degree from Queen's University in Canada.

C

Disclosure of Unavoidable
Conflicts of Interest

The conflict-of-interest policy of the National Academies of Sciences, Engineering, and Medicine (https://www.nationalacademies.org/about/institutional-policies-and-procedures/conflict-of-interest-policies-and-procedures) prohibits the appointment of an individual to a committee like the one that authored this consensus study report if the individual has a conflict of interest that is relevant to the task to be performed. An exception to this prohibition is permitted only if the National Academies determine that the conflict is unavoidable and the conflict is promptly and publicly disclosed.

When the committee that authored this report was established, a determination of whether there was a conflict of interest was made for each committee member given the individual's circumstances and the task being undertaken by the committee. A determination that an individual has a conflict of interest is not an assessment of that individual's actual behavior or character or ability to act objectively despite the conflicting interest.

Dr. Suma Babu has a financial conflict of interest because of her work as a physician investigator in industry-sponsored clinical trials of disease-modifying therapeutics for amyotrophic lateral sclerosis (ALS) supported by Biogen, Novartis, Ionis, OrphAI Therapeutics, and Denali. As of March 2024, she also serves as a compensated consultant for uniQure, a gene therapy company.

The National Academies have concluded that for this committee to accomplish the tasks for which it was established, its membership must include at least one individual with current leadership experience and expertise in clinical trials and expanded access programs involving industry sponsors. As described in her biographical summary, Dr. Babu bridges the interface between patient care and therapeutic development through her work at Massachusetts General Hospital leading a number of clinical trials and expanded access programs to benefit individuals living with ALS, with a particular focus on gene therapy, neuroimaging, and developing disease-modifying treatments and clinical trial biomarker readouts for patients with motor neuron diseases.

The National Academies have determined that the experience and expertise of Dr. Babu are needed for the committee to accomplish the task for which it has been established. The National Academies could not find another available individual with the equivalent experience and expertise who does not have a conflict of interest. Therefore, the National Academies have concluded that the conflict is unavoidable.

The National Academies believe that Dr. Babu can serve effectively as a member of the committee, and the committee can produce an objective report, taking into account the composition of the committee, the work to be performed, and the procedures to be followed in completing the study.

Dr. Chelsey R. Carter has a financial conflict of interest because of her work as a consultant on issues of race, equity, and inclusion for Amylyx, a pharmaceutical company developing new therapies for ALS.

The National Academies have concluded that for this committee to accomplish the tasks for which it was established, its membership must include at least one individual with current experience and expertise in race, equity, and inclusion and the experiences of people living with ALS. As described in her biographical summary, Dr. Carter brings significant experience and understanding of how systemic marginalization impacts historically underrepresented communities affected by neurodegenerative diseases, like ALS, and deep expertise in medicine, public health, and race. Dr. Carter is also undertaking a book project that includes an ethnographic study of the diverse experiences of living with ALS drawing on more than 15 years of experience with Black communities affected by ALS. Dr. Carter has previously been compensated for a presentation to Cytokinetics on issues of race, equity, and inclusion and currently presents on race, equity, and inclusion to Amylyx.

The National Academies have determined that the experience and expertise of Dr. Carter are needed for the committee to accomplish the task for which it has been established. The National Academies could not find another available individual with the equivalent experience and expertise who does not have a conflict of interest. Therefore, the National Academies have concluded that the conflict is unavoidable.

The National Academies believe that Dr. Carter can serve effectively as a member of the committee, and the committee can produce an objective report, taking into account the composition of the committee, the work to be performed, and the procedures to be followed in completing the study.

Dr. John Dunlop has a conflict of interest in relation to service on the Committee on Amyotrophic Lateral Sclerosis: Accelerating Treatments and Improving Quality of Life because of his relationships with Aliada Therapeutics, which develops therapeutics for central nervous system conditions including ALS.

The National Academies have concluded that for this committee to accomplish the tasks for which it was established, its membership must include at least one individual with current experience and expertise in private-sector ALS therapeutic research and development. As described in his biographical summary, Dr. Dunlop held scientific and leadership roles at firms such as Neumora Therapeutics, Amgen, AstraZeneca, Wyeth, and Pfizer, in addition to his current role as Chief Scientific Officer at Aliada. Dr. Dunlop also has ongoing roles for several entities and projects including the National Institutes of Health's HEAL Partnership Committee, Target-ALS, MassBio, Vigil Neuroscience, and the Packard Center for ALS Research at Johns Hopkins.

The National Academies have determined that the experience and expertise of Dr. Dunlop are needed for the committee to accomplish the task for which it has been established. The National Academies could not find another available individual with the equivalent experience and expertise who does not have a conflict of interest. Therefore, the National Academies have concluded that the conflict is unavoidable.

The National Academies believe that Dr. Dunlop can serve effectively as a member of the committee, and the committee can produce an objective report, taking into account the composition of the committee, the work to be performed, and the procedures to be followed in completing the study. In each case, the National Academies determined that the experience and expertise of the individual was needed for the committee to accomplish the task for which it was established. The National Academies could not find other available individuals who had the equivalent experience and expertise and did not have a conflict of interest. Therefore, the National Academies concluded that the conflicts were unavoidable and publicly disclosed them on its website (www.nationalacademies.org).